The Complete Pre-Dental Guide to Modern Dentistry

JOHN SYRBU

ISBN: 978-1468003413
ISBN-13: 1468003410

DEDICATION

This book is dedicated to my parents for their support, and my fiancé and friends in the Class of 2013 who helped make dental school a pleasant experience.

CONTENTS

NOTE FROM THE AUTHOR

This book is intended for the high school or college student with an interest in dentistry. Whether you've already been accepted into a dental program or are simply considering career options, this book will prove itself useful while shadowing dentists, during the interview process and well into dental school. My hope is that it provides you with a broad and basic understanding of the study and practice of dentistry. I've touched upon virtually every subject of most dental programs, and provided a foundation onto which your dental program will add many details.

Although the title mentions "modern practice," this book describes dentistry from a dental student's perspective. The views and opinions in this book are mine alone and do not necessarily reflect those of the University of Iowa College of Dentistry. As you will learn, dentistry is a field in which there are many different techniques, materials and philosophies based on your education, experience and location within the country.

I've also created a Facebook page called "The Complete Pre-Dental Guide to Modern Dentistry." I encourage comments and feedback in order to guide content and improve future editions. As a proponent of social media, the page may act as direct means of communication with the author as well as other readers.

Thank you for your readership, and I wish all of you the best of luck.

Your colleague,

John Syrbu
President, Class of 2013
University of Iowa
College of Dentistry

1

ASPECTS OF THE CAREER

There are many features and characteristics to the practice of dentistry, some of which you may have already come across in your consideration of the career. Before making a decision, it is advisable to converse with numerous dentists in order to gain several different perspectives. Depending on one's temperament, personal traits and previous experiences, dentistry may mean different things to different people. This chapter discusses several aspects that represent the career.

Providing a Service

Dental treatment provides a beneficial service to patients. Treatment can be as simple as an educational conversation teaching patients how to better care for their own teeth or as serious as diagnosing oral cancer. Dentists are considered primary care providers, and tend to see some patients more often than a physician. This makes it imperative that dentists not only know the oral cavity in great detail, but also be aware of many systemic diseases which have oral manifestations or require medical consultation. Though the road to dentistry may be long and at times strenuous, the self-fulfillment achieved from changing the lives of thousands of people in a beneficial way is irreplaceable.

The Dental Team

A dentist, even one who owns their own practice, works as part of a team to provide dental services to his or her patients. This "dental team" includes, but is not limited, to the dental assistant, the dental hygienist, a dental laboratory or dental technician, as well as the office staff of the practice.

Dental assistants integrate both interpersonal and technical skills, which greatly increase the efficiency and quality of the dental care provided to patients. Dental assistants primarily assist the dentist with a wide variety of procedures and seat patients to initiate the dental appointment. They may educate patients on proper oral hygiene techniques and give pre- and post-operative instructions to patients. Depending on the state and practice for which they work, their responsibilities may also include making dental radiographs, making impressions or sterilizing instruments and equipment.

Dental hygienists also work with dentists to provide patients with oral health care. Dental hygienists are known for their expertise in providing dental cleanings, commonly known among dentists as a "prophy," short for prophylaxis. They specialize in removing plaque and calculus (hard, mineralized plaque commonly known as tartar) from teeth, educating patients on oral hygiene and maintaining the health of the oral tissues. Other responsibilities of dental hygienists vary from state to state, but may include providing dental screenings such as an oral cancer screening, head and neck inspection and dental charting. Hygienists may also make radiographs and impressions and apply preventive materials such as fluoride and sealants, depending on the practice.

Developing a close relationship with a dental laboratory or a dental technician is imperative for a dental practice, especially for orthodontic and prosthodontic services. Dental technicians receive impressions or casts with detailed written instructions, known as a lab authorization, to fabricate a wide variety of appliances including crowns, bridges, dentures, veneers and orthodontic appliances. Dental technicians are experts at working with a variety of dental materials such as wax, plastics, metal alloys and a number of porcelains. With the help of a skilled dental technician, the dentist is able to deliver functional and attractive dental appliances to his or her patients.

The office staff is also an essential part of a patient's dental experience. It is important to have a friendly and pleasant staff to greet patients and make them feel comfortable as soon as they walk into the dental office. The attitude of the staff is reflective of how the office is run and can affect the initial perception of many patients. The staff is also usually in charge of scheduling and reminding patients of appointments either by phone, e-mail or postcard.

Dentistry: An Art and a Science

When people are unhappy with the appearance of their teeth they tend to smile less, which can have undue detriment to their self-esteem and emotional state. Dentists are trained to have the artistic and scientific knowledge and skill set needed to bring teeth to an esthetic shade and contour based on each patient's needs or desires. Teeth are important not only for eating and speaking but also function to maintain facial structure, support and appearance. An emphasis on the appearance of teeth is part of a branch of dentistry known as esthetic or cosmetic dentistry. The practical application of art and science is certainly an intriguing and rewarding aspect of dentistry that patients appreciate.

Dexterity in Dentistry

Dentistry is a very "hands-on" career and one that requires a considerable amount of dexterity coupled with an immense amount of scientific knowledge of the oral cavity and the body at large. Although some fields of dentistry exist which lessen the need for precise dexterity, such as Oral Pathology or Oral and Maxillofacial Radiology, all dental students must be competent with their hands in order to graduate and receive their license to practice dentistry. Whereas medical students graduate and may choose a residency or career path that requires dexterity, all dentists have a high level of dexterity upon graduating dental school and may practice as general dentists without a residency program of any sort. This is a key difference between medical and dental programs.

Variety is the Spice of Dentistry

The procedures we perform as dentists are as diverse as the patients we serve. Each patient is different and presents with different needs. Thus their treatment is tailored to their individual situation. Even within the same type of treatment, the etiology, presentation and method of treatment may all be varied. For example, dentists are commonly known to "drill-and-fill" cavities. These cavities, more precisely known as dental caries, may be on any tooth or root surface, may be at any stage in the caries process and may be treated with various different materials and methods. Dental caries is a single example of one of many oral diseases that a dentist can diagnose and help to treat. Simply put, there is no "one size fits all" approach to most dental treatment.

Furthermore, every patient is physically and emotionally distinct. Dentists have the opportunity to serve a large number of patients, often numbering in the thousands. The interpersonal variety that each patient brings to the practice makes dentistry an exciting career in which no day is like the previous one.

Autonomy and Flexibility

Dentists have the ability and privilege to own and manage their own practice. Whether starting a practice from the ground up, buying another dentist's practice or joining as a partner in a group, most dentists in the United States are employed in private practice. This autonomy allows a dentist to balance his or her professional and personal lives as they see fit, allowing them to choose not only when but also how they work. One can choose the materials they buy (the options are vast) and the equipment they use. To a certain extent, the general dentist may also gear his or her practice toward certain types of procedures by appealing to specific patient bases.

Lifelong Learning

At times, dental school can be demanding. The challenge of dentistry, however, is not limited to dental school but stays with the dentist well after graduation. Advancements in technology and material sciences are continuous, and dentists must stay informed on such topics by reading scientific magazines and attending continuing education (CE) courses and seminars throughout their careers. If you have an inherent interest in learning and seek a stimulating professional environment, dentistry will provide you with both of these amenities.

Ethics, Responsibility and Liability

All dentists are held to a high standard of ethics, as outlined by the ADA Principles of Ethics and Code of Professional Conduct. Although some patients experience anxiety toward dental visits, many people trust the dentist to provide them honest and balanced advice and treatment. Some core values and principles that make dentistry the trusted and respected profession it is today are summarized below:

Autonomy

The dentist must preserve the patient's rights to participate in self-determination and respect patient confidentiality. Patients should be informed of the treatment options and should be involved with treatment decisions while maintaining confidentiality between the dentist and the patient.

Nonmaleficence

The dentist has the responsibility to "do no harm" to the patient. For example, if a general dentist is not comfortable or competent with complex root canal treatments, it is best for them to refer the patient to an endodontist.

Beneficence

The dentist must act in the patient's best interest and welfare. From the previous example, it is in the patient's best interest to be treated by the dental specialist rather than their regular dentist.

Justice

The dentist should treat patients fairly and equally. A dentist provides oral health care regardless of a patient's race, background or belief and standardizes their treatment to avoid any interferences of this sort.

Veracity

The dentist must communicate truthfully and honestly with the patient concerning all aspects of treatment. Mistakes can and will happen, and dentists are people too. An even bigger mistake is not informing the patient when critical errors occur.

These codes of conduct will be reiterated within the dental curriculum and tested in classes as well as on board examinations. Not only are these ethical principles important to follow on a personal and professional level, but they often prove to be important from a legal aspect. In a litigious society, patients have the right to bring their dentist to court if they feel that the dentist has acted wrongfully. Most patients are very understanding of mistakes when they are informed of such occurrences. Practitioners who try to hide critical errors experience less compassion from their patients, which can lead to litigation. Abiding closely to ethical codes, informing patients throughout the treatment process and building a trusting relationship with patients provides the best protection from legal actions even in the unfortunate event of a mistake or misunderstanding.

Earning potential: A Factor, not a Determinant

The earning potential of dentistry can be both a practical consideration and a lucrative attraction. Dentists continually earn average incomes in the top 5% of

U.S. family incomes. While this can be a factor in the consideration for a career path, it should not be the deciding factor.

It is also important to consider the cost of a dental education. Dental students accumulate an average student loan debt of roughly $200,000 upon graduation. Those who are not truly passionate about dentistry will likely find dental school unbearable and struggle to find fulfillment. Thus, the earning potential of this prestigious career should be secondary to a deeper passion for the practice of dentistry.

2

OPPORTUNITIES IN DENTISTRY

Just as the term "medicine" is fairly vague, the term "dentistry" encompasses a wide variety of ideas and aspects of an exciting field of study and practice. In addition to general dentistry, there are nine formally recognized dental specialties. After choosing between general dentistry and a specialty, the majority of dentists will choose to work in private practice, either alone or as an associate in a group practice. Some opt for a career in academic dentistry or public service. The military provides employment opportunities as well as loan repayment programs. Dental research also provides many opportunities for dentists as a profession in itself or as part of an academic career. A relatively new option for dentists is to work for a franchise in which a company finances and manages a practice, relieving the dentist of these duties. Numerous dental organizations exist, at the local and national level, for both general dentistry and dental specialties. There are also many opportunities for dentists to volunteer their services which offer a very rewarding experience.

General Dentistry vs. Dental Specialty

The field of dentistry currently consists of general dentistry as well as nine dental specialties formally recognized by the American Dental Association (www.ada.org). While most of the roughly 180,000 practicing dentists in the United States are general practitioners, about twenty percent are dental specialists. Definitions of the nine dental specialties approved by the Council on Dental Education and Licensure are as follows:

Dental Public Health

Dental public health is the science and art of preventing and controlling dental diseases and promoting dental health through organized community efforts. It is that form of dental practice which serves the community as a patient rather than the individual. It is concerned with the dental health education of the public, with applied dental research, and with the administration of group dental care programs as well as the prevention and control of dental diseases on a community basis. (Adopted May 1976)

Endodontics

Endodontics is the branch of dentistry which is concerned with the morphology, physiology and pathology of the human dental pulp and periradicular tissues. Its study and practice encompass the basic and clinical sciences including biology of the normal pulp, the etiology, diagnosis, prevention and treatment of diseases and injuries of the pulp and associated periradicular conditions. (Adopted December 1983)

Oral and Maxillofacial Pathology

Oral pathology is the specialty of dentistry and discipline of pathology that deals with the nature, identification, and management of diseases affecting the oral and maxillofacial regions. It is a science that investigates the causes, processes, and effects of these diseases. The practice of oral pathology includes research and diagnosis of diseases using clinical, radiographic, microscopic, biochemical, or other examinations. (Adopted May 1991)

Oral and Maxillofacial Radiology

Oral and maxillofacial radiology is the specialty of dentistry and discipline of radiology concerned with the production and interpretation of images and data produced by all modalities of radiant energy that are used for the diagnosis and management of diseases, disorders and conditions of the oral and maxillofacial region. (Adopted April 2001)

Oral and Maxillofacial Surgery

Oral and maxillofacial surgery is the specialty of dentistry which includes the diagnosis, surgical and adjunctive treatment of diseases, injuries and defects involving both the functional and esthetic aspects of the hard and soft tissues of the oral and maxillofacial region. (Adopted October 1990)

Orthodontics and Dentofacial Orthopedics

Orthodontics and dentofacial orthopedics is the dental specialty that includes the diagnosis, prevention, interception, and correction of malocclusion, as well as neuromuscular and skeletal abnormalities of the developing or mature orofacial structures. (Adopted April 2003)

Pediatric Dentistry

Pediatric Dentistry is an age-defined specialty that provides both primary and comprehensive preventive and therapeutic oral health care for infants and children through adolescence, including those with special health care needs. (Adopted 1995)

Periodontics

Periodontics is that specialty of dentistry which encompasses the prevention, diagnosis and treatment of diseases of the supporting and surrounding tissues of the teeth or their substitutes and the maintenance of the health, function and esthetics of these structures and tissues. (Adopted December 1992)

Prosthodontics

Prosthodontics is the dental specialty pertaining to the diagnosis, treatment planning, rehabilitation and maintenance of the oral function, comfort, appearance and health of patients with clinical conditions associated with missing or deficient teeth and/or oral and maxillofacial tissues using biocompatible substitutes. (Adopted April 2003)

Private practice

Upon deciding between general dentistry and a dental specialty, most dentists enter private practice and work either in a solo practice or in partnerships with other dentists. While starting a practice from the ground up is an option, many graduates find employment as an associate in an established practice. With a large number of retiring dentists, graduates may transition into a practice with a dentist phasing to retirement.

Academics and careers in Public Service

Loan repayment is a considerable factor for recent graduates. Most federally-funded academic positions offer some sort of loan repayment assistance, such as those that qualify for the Public Service Loan Forgiveness Program. Academic positions usually combine teaching, research, community service and patient care. While academic dentists tend to earn less income on a yearly basis, the work benefits and intellectually stimulating environment of academic dentistry are nearly unmatched.

Private practice and academia are not necessarily mutually exclusive. Dentists have the option to work in their private practice some days of the week and at a teaching institution as adjunct faculty, teaching as much or as little as they desire.

Other government-related careers are available to dentists, such as the Indian Health Service (www.ihs.gov) or many community health centers. A contract for several years of service usually offers yearly loan repayment in addition to a base salary. Rural or underserved areas in need of dentists may also provide a sign-on bonus and loan repayment benefits.

Service in the Federal Government

Several opportunities exist for dental graduates through the military. The Army, Navy and Air Force enlists dentists to provide oral health care to military personnel and their families. As part of a federal program, the military also offers many scholarships and loan repayment options for those who participate.

Dental Research

Dental research is an invigorating field which continually influences the scope and direction of dentistry. Dental techniques and treatment methods are guided by Evidence-Based Dentistry (ebd.ada.org), the idea that the practice of dentistry should be based on the latest research findings. Evidence-Based Dentistry measures the strength of information gained from each study or experiment. For example, a randomized clinical trial will provide stronger evidence than a retrospective study that relies heavily on patient records.

Advancements in technology also play a major role in virtually all aspects of modern dentistry. From a new device used in the diagnosis of oral disease to an improved restorative material providing stronger adhesion to tooth structure, technology continues to drive dentistry forward. Dentists can keep up with advancements by enrolling in continuing education (CE) courses, attending conferences and reading scientific journals such as the Journal of the American Dental Association (JADA).

Franchised Dental Practices

A relatively new trend in dentistry is on the rise, commonly referred to as franchised or "chain" dentistry. When compared to private practitioners, who assume all aspects of their practice including business endeavors, a chain or franchise that owns a practice will run the practice, per se. Essentially, dental chains act to free dentists of the business and management responsibilities of owning a practice, allowing the dentist to focus primarily on treating patients. For example, a company may purchase a practice from a retiring dentist, buy all necessary supplies, hire personnel and continue to manage the practice, leaving the dentist with the sole responsibility of treating patients. This mode of practice may limit the practitioner in various ways, thus the terms and conditions of the contract should be taken into careful consideration by the dentist.

This model for dental practice may be particularly appealing for new dentists. Recent graduates can focus on building skill and efficiency while reducing the weight of running a practice. This option may also be financially attractive, as buying a practice or starting one from scratch can be quite expensive. Thus, a franchised practice may facilitate a reasonable income more quickly.

Organized Dentistry

Organized dentistry encompasses many organizations that provide structure and work to improve and advance the dental profession. Each organization caters to a specific group of dentists within the various fields of dentistry, and each is governed and lead by dentists. At least one organization exists for each of the dental specialties and numerous other groups within the field of dentistry. Each organization requires a fee for membership and in turn offers different member benefits, such as advocating in their interest. Most organizations host annual meetings which provide information and networking opportunities.

Some organizations offer discounted rates for dental students. The organization that represents dental students is the American Student Dental Association (ASDA), which is affiliated with the American Dental Association

(ADA). ASDA members receive a number of benefits, from monthly publications of the Journal of the American Dental Association (JADA) to free life insurance. As a member of ASDA, and in turn the ADA, you are a part of the tri-partite system, and thus a member at the local, state and national level. ASDA also hosts annual district, regional and national meetings that leaders and members have the opportunity to attend.

Volunteering

Only about 50% of the United States population has dental insurance. Some are not able to afford dental treatment while others may reside in an area where adequate dental services are simply not available to them. Many people are faced with these difficulties worldwide. Volunteering as a dentist not only provides you with an incredibly rewarding experience, but provides people with a valuable service. Fortunately, there are many organizations which provide the opportunity for both dentists as well as dental students to participate in service trips. Some are led by dentists while others by physicians. Regardless of the leadership, these organizations work for a very worthy cause in which many dentists choose to participate throughout their careers.

3

BASIC DENTAL ANATOMY AND TERMINOLOGY

Many professionals use technical terminology catered to their specific area of expertise. The dental profession is no exception. The dentist normally explains things to his or her patient in "common language" to ensure a basic understanding and then switches to a "dental language" when discussing things amongst other dentists or dental personnel such as the assistant or the hygienist. This section will help make sense of commonly used dental terms through a brief study of dental anatomy and descriptive terminology.

The Maxilla and Mandible

Human teeth are arranged in two opposing arches within the upper and lower jaws. Teeth in the upper jaw are known as maxillary teeth, because they are housed within the maxilla, while the lower teeth are termed mandibular teeth and housed within the mandible or lower jaw. In Figure 3.1, the maxilla is depicted in blue and the mandible in orange.

To standardize orientation and communication, dentists divide the face and head along several imaginary planes. The most common reference plane is the midline of the face, extending vertically along the middle of the nose through the middle two maxillary teeth. This imaginary plane running through the midline to the back of the head is called the mid-sagittal plane (Figure 3.2). The maxillary and mandibular arches are divided equally by this plane, resulting in four quadrants of the mouth: the maxillary (upper) right, maxillary left, mandibular (lower) right and mandibular left. Two other imaginary planes are used for orientation, one running horizontally, appropriately named the horizontal plane, and the other sectioning the head lengthwise through the ears, called the frontal or coronal plane. It is also important to remember that when a dentist looks directly at a patient, the patient's right and left are reversed in reference to the dentist. When referring to a patient, a dentist will always use the patient's anatomical references, i.e. their right and left.

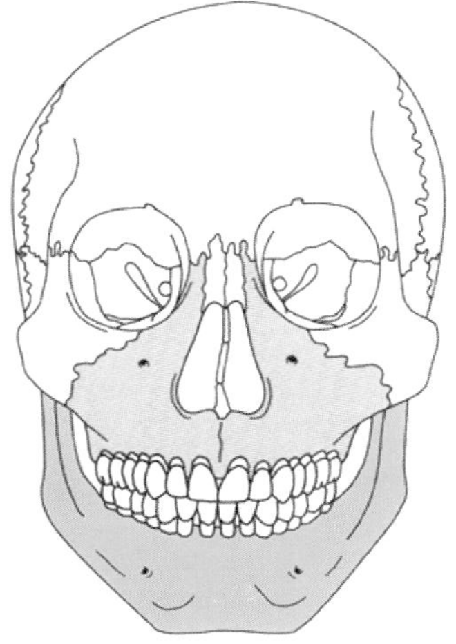

Figure 3.1 A human skull highlighting the maxilla (blue) and the mandible (orange) which house the upper and lower teeth, respectively.

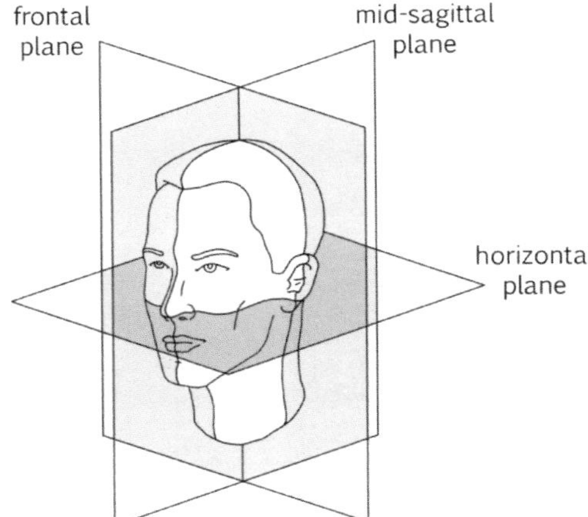

Figure 3.2 The head is sectioned along three imaginary planes: the mid-sagittal plane, horizontal plane and frontal or coronal plane.

The Temporomandibular Joint (TMJ)

One of the most important joints in dentistry is the temporomandibular joint, or TMJ, which allows one to open and close their mouth. As the name implies, these two joints unite the temporal bones of the skull with the mandible. Anatomically, the joint is located just anterior to the ears and may be palpated and assessed by placing two fingers just anterior to the ears while the patient opens and closes their mouth.

Primary, Mixed and Permanent Dentitions

Humans have two separate sets of teeth, or dentitions: the deciduous, or primary dentition and the adult, or permanent dentition. Dentitions can also be grouped in three different phases: the primary dentition phase, the mixed dentition phase and the permanent dentition phase. The first set, nicknamed "baby teeth," are formally known as primary or deciduous dentition, so named because they shed like leaves of deciduous trees. With the eruption of the permanent mandibular central incisors, a child of about 6 years will enter the mixed or transitional phase, which is when both primary and permanent teeth are present in the mouth. All primary teeth are eventually shed (formally termed "exfoliation"), and replaced by permanent teeth. A child will enter the permanent dentition phase at around age 12 with the exfoliation of his or her primary second molars.

Primary Dentition

Deciduous or primary dentition is further discussed in Pediatric Dentistry and Orthodontics (Chapter 8).

Permanent Dentition

There are normally a total of 32 permanent teeth. The permanent dentition consists of 8 incisors, 4 canines, 8 premolars and 12 molars (Figure 3.3). In general, mandibular teeth tend to erupt before their maxillary counterparts and begin with the mandibular central incisors at about 6 years of age. Permanent first molars, or "6 year molars," commonly erupt simultaneously with mandibular central incisors and come in behind primary second molars. After all incisors have erupted, the mandibular canines erupt, followed by the mandibular first premolars and then the maxillary first premolars. The maxillary canines tend to erupt around the time that the second premolars erupt and may even erupt after them. Permanent second molars, often referred to as "12 year molars," erupt next, followed by third molars, or "wisdom teeth," about five to nine years later.

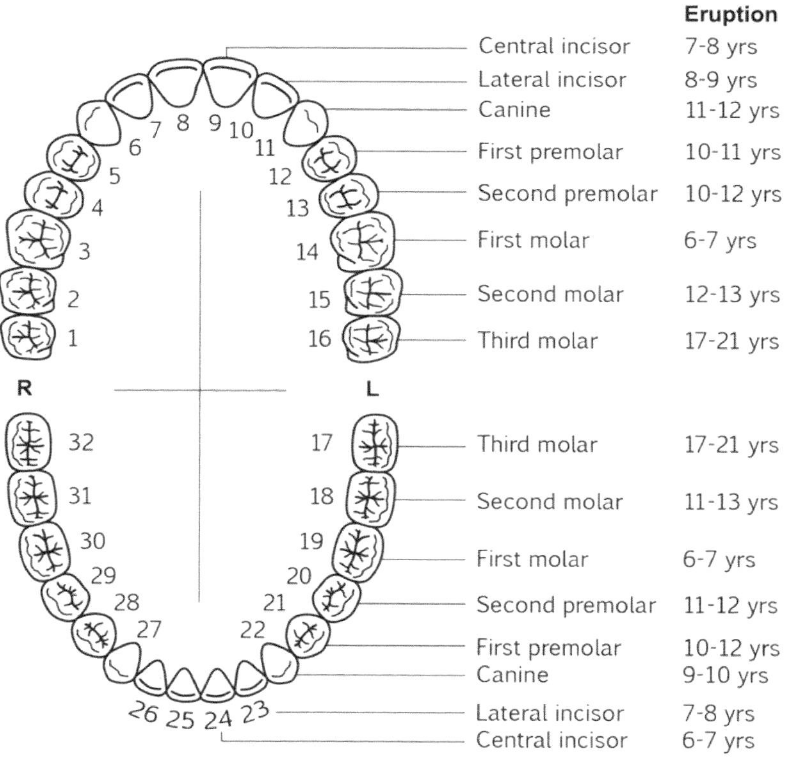

Figure 3.3 The universal numbering system and eruption sequence of permanent dentition.

Universal Numbering System

Although there are several systems for numbering teeth, the universal system is most widely used (hence the name). The system assigns a number to each of the permanent teeth (1-32), starting with the upper right third molar and counts leftward from 1 to 16, the maxillary left third molar. The system then drops down to the mandibular left third molar, #17, and counts rightward to the mandibular right third molar, #32 (Figure 3.3). A good way to recall which number is assigned to a given tooth is to remember certain teeth and count from them, for example the maxillary centrals are right to left, #8 and #9, while the mandibular centrals are left to right, #24 and #25. Other people remember the canines as #6, #11, #22 and #27 and count left or right from them. While it takes some practice to master, the universal numbering system is widely used in dentistry and speeds up communication considerably.

The numbering system for deciduous teeth is discussed in Chapter 8, Pediatric Dentistry and Orthodontics.

Anterior teeth

Anterior teeth are those in the front of the mouth and include the incisors and canines. They function in mastication to bite, incise, cut and shear. Anterior teeth are also essential in phonetics and esthetics. They reside in what is considered the "esthetic zone" which is normally visible when people speak and smile.

Posterior teeth

The teeth in the back of the mouth are considered posterior teeth, and include the premolars and molars. Their main function in mastication is grinding, and to a lesser extent also function in esthetics and phonetics.

The Tooth

Each tooth consists of crown and root portions. Hard tissues of the tooth include enamel and dentin, which surround a soft pulp that supplies nutrients and sensory innervation to each tooth.

Crown (Anatomical vs. Clinical)

The anatomical crown is the portion of the tooth covered by enamel while the clinical crown is the part of the tooth that is visible when one looks in the mouth (Figure 3.4). These two entities do not necessarily correspond, depending on the level of the gums. For example, with a receding gumline, the clinical crown may include part of the exposed root surface. Thus the clinical crown is not a constant entity like the anatomical crown.

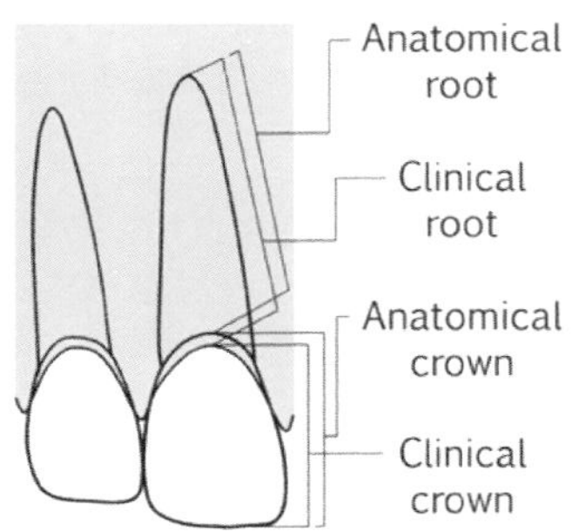

Figure 3.4 Each tooth has one crown and up to three roots. The anatomical crown and root depend on the limits of the enamel, whereas the clinical crown and root depend on what is visible in the mouth.

Root (Anatomical vs. Clinical)

The root of the tooth may also be anatomical or clinical. The anatomical root refers to the portion of the tooth that is covered by cementum, a thin mineralized tissue further discussed under "The Periodontium" section of this chapter. The clinical root is complimentary to the clinical crown, and is defined as the portion of the tooth which is not visible (Figure 3.4). Similarly, the clinical root may change throughout life while the anatomical root is a constant entity.

Enamel

Enamel is composed of about 96% inorganic salts, 3% water and 1% organic proteins by weight. The inorganic component is a hexagonal crystalline lattice called hydroxyapatite [$Ca_{10}(PO_4)_6(OH)_2$] which aligns to form elongated rods. These rods are oriented more or less perpendicular to the crown surface and parallel to each other (Figure 3.5). As the hardest tissue in the body, enamel functions to protect the underlying dentin and pulp. Conversely, enamel's integrity relies on sound underlying dentin for shock absorption, as enamel itself is otherwise quite brittle and susceptible to fracture.

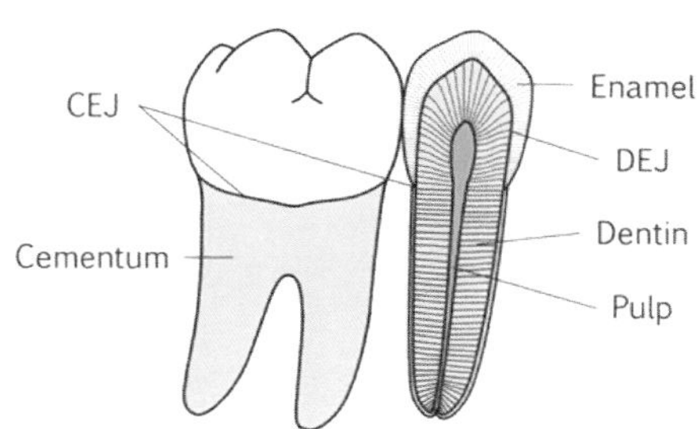

Figure 3.5 The outer surface of the anatomical crown is covered by enamel and the root by a thin layer of cementum. The junction of these two layers is known as the cemento-enamel junction (CEJ). Inside these layers is a thicker layer of dentin which encloses the pulp. The internal junction of the dentin with the enamel is appropriately named the dentino-enamel junction (DEJ).

Dentin and the DEJ

Dentin is the second hardest tissue in the body. It is composed of roughly 70% inorganic hydroxyapatite, 20% organic proteins and 10% water by weight. Comparable to enamel rods, dentin's structure is comprised of S-shaped dentinal tubules that extend from the enamel to the pulp. The internal junction of the dentin and the enamel within the anatomical crown is known as the dentino-enamel junction or DEJ (Figure 3.5).

The Pulp

Dental pulp is the innermost portion of the tooth and provides a vital (living) tooth with nutrients via blood vessels and sensory innervation via nerves. Unlike dentin and enamel, pulp is gel-like in consistency and composed of about 75% water and 25% organic materials. The pulp also contains living cells which synthesize and deposit dentin throughout life, known as secondary dentin, which effectively reduces the size of the pulp cavity as one ages. Dentin synthesis and deposition is also increased locally in response to bacterial infiltration. This type of dentin is known as reparative or tertiary dentin (Figure 3.6).

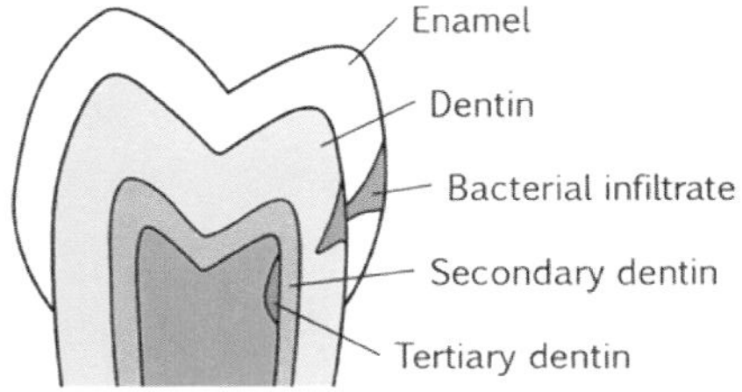

Figure 3.6 The pulp is contained within the dentin of a tooth. A dynamic entity, pulp continually deposits secondary dentin throughout life. Tertiary dentin may be deposited locally in response to bacterial offense.

Components of the Pulp Cavity

The pulp cavity of a tooth refers to the entire internal space in which the pulp resides. The pulp cavity is composed of a pulp chamber, pulp horn(s) and one to several pulp canals. The pulp chamber is the swollen part of the pulp cavity contained mostly within the crown of the tooth. Pulp chambers often follow the contours of the crown, and when they extend upward with the cusps of teeth, the extensions of the pulp chambers are known as pulp horns. Pulp canals are the portions of the pulp cavity which extend into the root(s) of the tooth (Figure 3.7).

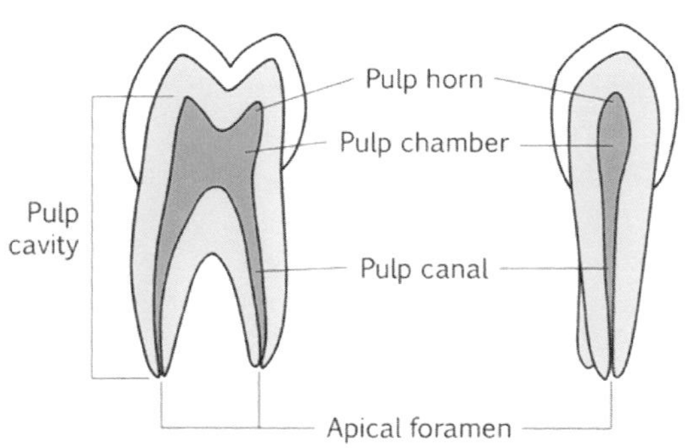

Figure 3.7 The pulp cavity contains the pulp tissue of each tooth. The pulp chamber is the bulbous part of the pulp cavity within the crown of the tooth. Pulp horns are cusp-like occlusal or incisal extensions of the pulp chamber while pulp canals reside within and extend to the apex of each root. Blood vessels and nerves supply the tooth by entering through the apical foramen of each root tip.

The periodontium

The periodontium is the general name given to the hard and soft supporting tissues of the teeth (Figure 3.8) and include the following:

Cementum and the CEJ

Cementum is a thin layer of mineralized avascular tissue which covers the anatomical root of the tooth (see Figure 3.5). The mineral is also hydroxyapatite with a slightly larger proportion of organic matrix than dentin, making it somewhat softer than dentin. The main function of the cementum is to act as the attachment apparatus of the tooth to the bone via fibers of the periodontal ligament (PDL). The junction of the anatomical crown with the root, or where enamel meets cementum, is called the cemento-enamel junction, or CEJ. The CEJ acts as a point of reference, for example when the gums recede past the CEJ to expose the root surface, it is considered gingival recession.

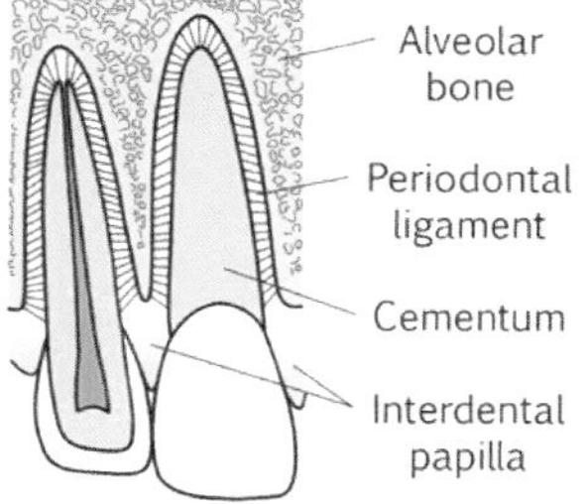

Figure 3.8 Teeth are suspended within alveoli by the periodontal ligament, which attaches to cementum and alveolar bone. Alveolar bone is covered by fibrous gingiva which normally extends between teeth, where it is termed interdental papilla.

Periodontal Ligament (PDL)

The periodontal ligament, or PDL, is the fibrous tissue which attaches the tooth to its socket within the maxilla or mandible. The PDL fibers of the PDL consist mainly of collagen and connect to the cementum at one end and alveolar bone at the other.

The Alveolar Process

Two alveolar processes exist: the alveolar process of the maxilla and that of the mandible. These are the portions of each respective bone that house the teeth of each dental arch. Each tooth is contained within a socket, or alveolus, and there are normally 16 alveoli within each alveolar process (further discussed in Chapter 10). The unique joint type between a tooth, the fibrous periodontal ligament and its alveolus is known as a gomphosis joint.

Gingiva

What is commonly referred to as "gums" is more accurately described as gingiva. Gingiva is the fibrous tissue covered by a mucous membrane that attaches to the alveolar bone and to individual teeth.

Interdental papilla

Interdental papillae (pl.) are the portions of the gingiva that extend between teeth (interproximally), viewed from the facial as triangles between the gingival thirds of teeth.

Coronal Surfaces

Each tooth crown has five surfaces: one surface is towards the midline, one away from the midline, one towards the lips or cheeks, one towards the tongue or palate and a biting surface that contacts teeth in the opposing arch. For all teeth, the surface towards the midline is known as the mesial surface. The opposite surface facing away from the midline is known as the distal surface. It should also be noted that the area between teeth is known as the interproximal area. The surface on the inside of the mouth facing the tongue is known as the lingual surface, or sometimes called the palatal surface for maxillary teeth. For anterior teeth, the outside surface contacting the lips is termed the labial surface (Figure 3.9a), while for posterior teeth it is referred to as the buccal surface because it contacts the cheek, or buccal mucosa (3.9b). Alternatively, the labial or buccal surfaces for all teeth may also be referred to as the facial surface. The biting surfaces also differ for anterior and posterior teeth. For anterior teeth, the surface is more of an edge and termed the incisal edge, while posterior teeth have a developed chewing surface known as the occlusal surface.

Additionally, the area close to the CEJ is referred to as the cervix (neck) or cervical area of the tooth, because teeth circumferentially constrict slightly about the CEJ. The CEJ tends to coincide with the gingival margin and thus cervical and gingival may be interchangeable. It should be noted that these designations are not limited to single tooth crowns but can be used as descriptive terms when referring to a quadrant as a whole (Figure 3.10).

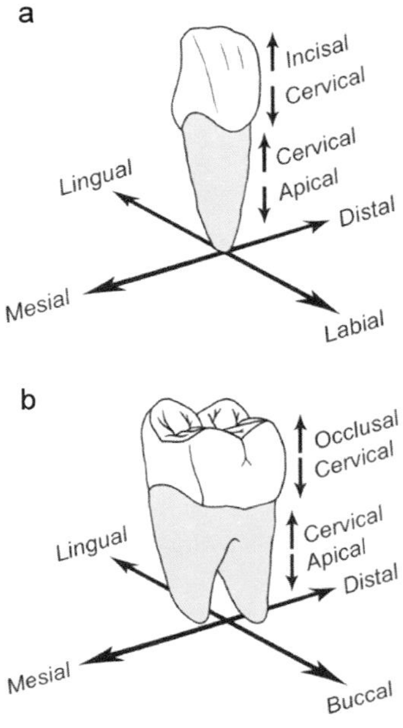

Figure 3.9 Descriptive terminology for anterior (a) and posterior teeth (b). Note that the facial tooth surface is referred to as "labial" for anterior teeth and "buccal" for posterior teeth, and "incisal" equates to "occlusal".

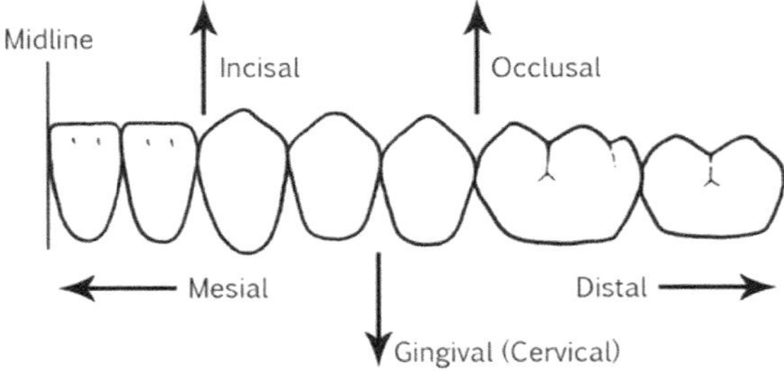

Figure 3.10 The same terminology can be used when referring to multiple teeth or a whole quadrant.

Coronal Structure

Each tooth type has characteristic anatomical features with many variations from person to person. As a sample reference tooth, we will discuss some of the coronal features of tooth #3, the permanent maxillary right first molar (Figure 3.11a). This tooth has four cusps which make up most of the occlusal surface of the tooth (3.12b). Premolars, also known as bicuspids, have two cusps while canines, or cuspids, have just one. Incisors do not possess cusps. Pits and grooves are also found on the occlusal surfaces of posterior teeth and lingual surfaces of anterior teeth. A discontinuous groove runs across the occlusal surfaces of all posterior teeth in a mesiodistal direction, known on each as the central groove. The maxillary right first molar also possesses a buccal groove that extends from the central groove onto the buccal surface as well as a lingual groove that extends onto the lingual surface. Small depressions where grooves begin, join or terminate are known as pits (3.11c). Molars possess mesial, central and distal pits while premolars only have mesial and distal pits. Pits and grooves sometimes appear on the lingual surfaces of anterior teeth as well.

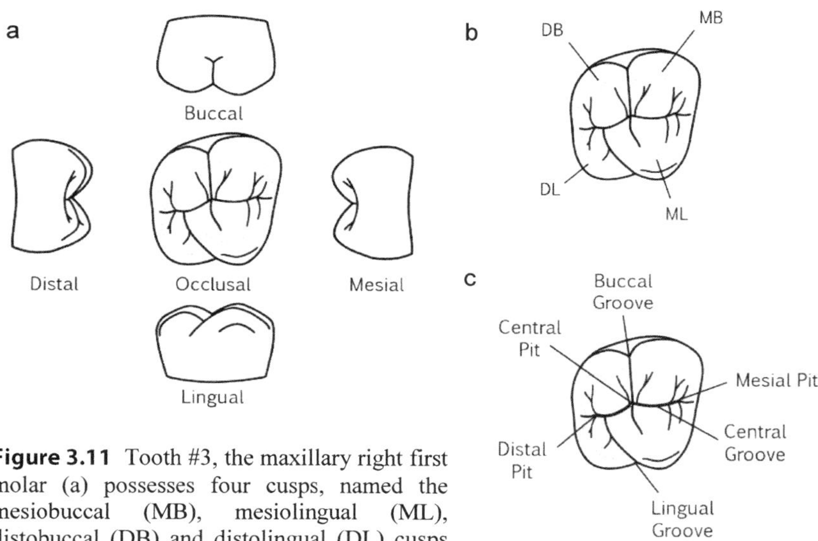

Figure 3.11 Tooth #3, the maxillary right first molar (a) possesses four cusps, named the mesiobuccal (MB), mesiolingual (ML), distobuccal (DB) and distolingual (DL) cusps (b). Several depressions such as pits and grooves also exist on the occlusal surface (c).

Root Surfaces

Axial root surface designations (i.e. mesial, distal, lingual and facial) are the same as for the crown, however roots lack an incisal or occlusal surface (Figure 3.9). Instead, the coronal limit of the root is the CEJ and areas of the root surrounding the CEJ are also considered to be cervical. At the tip of each root is an opening known as the apical foramen (see Figure 3.7). The apical foramen serves as a pore through which blood vessels and sensory nerves reach the pulp of the tooth, and is thus said to be towards the apical portion of the root.

4

CARIOLOGY AND DENTAL PUBLIC HEALTH

Compared to other specialties, the patient of a public health dentist is the community rather than the individual. A public health dentist works to prevent and control dental decay and to promote oral health in general through community efforts. A Master's in Dental Public Health may emphasize topics such as health planning and administration, biostatistics, epidemiology and environmental health. Public health dentists are then employed at the federal, state and local level and at educational institutions as well as in the private sector. More information may be obtained from the American Association of Public Health Dentistry (http://www.aaphd.org).

Public health initiatives may be accomplished through assessment, policy development and assurance. Assessment refers to regularly and systematically collecting and analyzing data on the health of a community, for example statistics on health status and community needs. Public health dentistry then promotes the use of scientific knowledge gained during the assessment phase in order to develop public health policy, such as school-based dental screening programs for children. Public health agencies must also assure its constituents that the services necessary to meet the community needs are being provided. This may be in the form of a monitoring system or an assessment of the needs some time after a policy is implemented.

All dental programs include content on dental public health, as all dentists have a role in diagnosing and treating dental disease within their communities.

Etiology of Caries

For as long as humans have had teeth, tooth decay has existed. Dental caries is still one of the most prevalent chronic diseases worldwide. A distinction must be made between dental caries and "cavities". Dental caries is the disease process in which the metabolic byproducts of microorganisms result in a progressive destruction of tooth structure. In other words, caries is the process from which cavitation may result, however decay occurs along a continuum and need not be cavitated.

Four main components interact to produce caries: tooth structure, microorganisms, a substrate and adequate time for the interaction to take place (Figure 4.1). Tooth structure must be present, namely enamel or dentin, to which certain bacteria adhere. Although several microorganisms have been associated with dental decay, a key contributor to caries is the species *Streptococcus Mutans*, a gram-positive coccus. In general, microorganisms capable of producing decay, termed cariogenic bacteria, are those that metabolize fermentable sugars to produce acidic byproducts. These acidic metabolites then dissolve or demineralize tooth structure and eventually result in a "cavity".

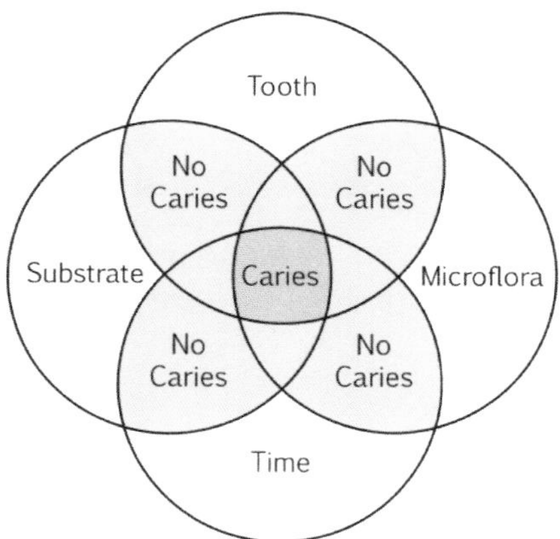

Figure 4.1 Four components interact to produce caries. Without one, dental decay does not occur.

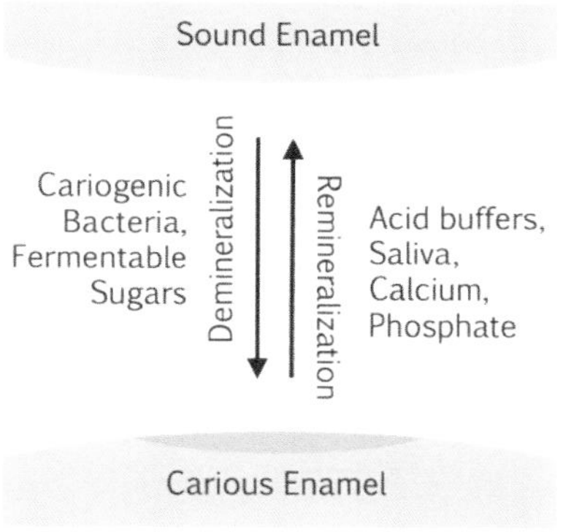

Figure 4.2 Various factors contribute to the "push-and-pull" equilibrium that exists between demineralization and remineralization at the tooth surface.

As mentioned in Chapter 3, enamel and dentin are largely composed of inorganic salts in a lattice known as hydroxyapatite $[Ca_{10}(PO_4)_6(OH)_2]$. A dynamic equilibrium exists in the oral cavity at the surface of the tooth in which adherent bacteria produce acidic metabolites to demineralize or dissolve sound enamel into carious enamel. Alternatively, acid buffers or mineral salts such as calcium and phosphate can reverse this process and remineralize the tooth to produce sound enamel (Figure 4.2). Once bacteria have dissolved enough enamel to reach the dentin, they may travel through the dentinal tubules to reach the pulp at an accelerated rate.

Detection and Diagnosis of Caries

Diagnosing dental caries takes some experience and combines several forms of detection. Before even looking in the mouth, a dentist can interview the patient to estimate their caries risk. For example, a patient history including dietary habits, oral hygiene practices, smoking status and a list of current medications are all necessary for an evaluation. A clinical examination of the mouth requires clean, dry teeth for proper assessment. Radiographic images also aid in detecting decay, especially on interproximal surfaces where teeth contact each other. A probe or an explorer is also commonly used as a tactile adjunct to determine the texture of a lesion. Carious tooth structure will "catch" or "stick" an explorer in the lesion.

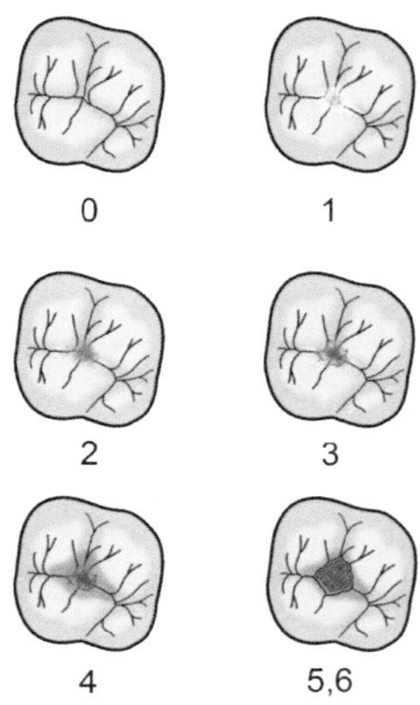

Figure 4.3 The International Caries Detection and Assessment System (ICDAS).

Numerous classification systems exist to detect and classify carious lesions. A system recently developed by researchers from the United Kindgom, the United States and Europe is known as the International Caries Detection and Assessment System (ICDAS, Figure 4.3). This system scores carious lesions from "0" to "6" based on their extent and severity. A score of "0" is sound enamel with no evidence of caries and no change after air-drying the tooth for five seconds. A "1" is the first visual change in enamel where the lesion cannot be seen at first but appears white or brown upon air-drying for five seconds. A lesion with a score of "2" is distinct and can be visualized without air-drying. Lesions with a score of "3" present with localized breakdown of the enamel surface but without visible dentin. A score of "4" is given to non-cavitated lesions with an underlying blue/grey/brown shadowing from the affected underlying dentin. Scores of "5" and "6" are reserved for distinctly cavitated lesions with moderate or extensive dentin visible, respectively.

Sealants

A large component of dental public health emphasizes the prevention of caries. In particular with susceptible occlusal anatomy, i.e. deep pits and fissures, a dentist need not wait and watch for carries to occur. A sealant, unlike a conventional restoration, is placed in the occlusal pits and fissures of a tooth as a preventive measure, before any dental decay has occurred (Figure 4.4). Microscopically, many pits and fissures are deep enough that they house bacterial colonies and narrow enough that a tooth brush bristle cannot penetrate to its depth, thus making it hard to cleanse and susceptible to caries. As long as the pit or fissure is well-sealed, a more favorable anatomy is created which is more cleansable and less likely to trap bacteria. In young children especially, the practice of sealant placement is an effective way to prevent dental decay. Many school-based sealant programs have been created as a dental public health initiative in which dentists and dental hygienists place sealants.

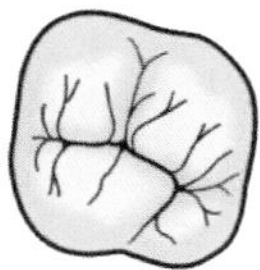
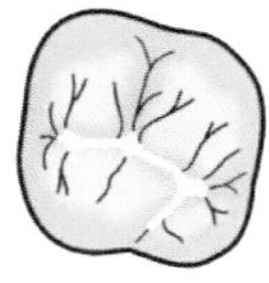

Figure 4.4 Deep occlusal pits and fissures can be maintained by placing sealants.

To place a sealant, the tooth or teeth are isolated, cleaned and rinsed with water. The enamel is then etched with acid, rinsed again with water and dried completely. The sealant, commonly a light-activated bis-GMA epoxy resin, is applied and light-cured.

The Role of Fluoride, Water Fluoridation and Fluorosis

The effects of fluoride were first recognized by dentists in mountainous regions with naturally high water fluoride content. Dentists in these regions noted that teeth tended to present with more staining, an observation affectionately known as "Colorado brown stain" from where it originated, and also tended to experience fewer caries. Researchers later discovered several mechanisms by which fluoride acts to reduce caries, such as the promotion of remineralization and inhibition of a key enzyme in the bacterial metabolism of glucose known as enolase.

Community water fluoridation refers to the adjustment of fluoride in drinking water to optimal levels (about 1 part per million) as a preventive measure in order to reduce the incidence of caries. Since 1945, when Grand Rapids, Michigan became the first city to fluoridate its water supply, studies have consistently shown that water fluoridation is both safe and effective. In fact, the Center for Disease Control (CDC) has deemed water fluoridation as one of the top ten greatest public health accomplishments of the 20th century (http://www.cdc.gov/fluoridation).

At higher-than-optimal fluoride concentration, enamel staining may occur. This condition, known as fluorosis, appears as faint white streaks on enamel surfaces. Teeth exposed to even higher concentrations during their development may experience moderate to severe enamel fluorosis, appearing as brown staining with a mottled appearance. However, fluorosis can only occur when primary or permanent teeth are developing. Once teeth have erupted, fluorosis is no longer a risk.

5

GENERAL DENTISTRY AND RESTORATIVE PROCEDURES

General dentistry is the field in which most dentists practice. Upon graduation, a dental student receives either a Doctor of Dental Surgery (D.D.S) or Doctor of Dental Medicine (D.M.D.) degree and may start working as a general dentist. Residency programs are also an option for graduating students to gain experience prior to practice, such as the Advanced Education in General Dentistry (AEGD) or the General Practice Residency (GPR). Several organizations represent general dentistry and may provide additional information, such as the Academy of General Dentistry (www.agd.org).

Once in practice, a general dentist provides a wide variety of services to patients. For example, a general dentist very commonly provides prosthetic services such as crowns or simple orthodontic services to children. General dentists may also provide more complex treatments such as implant therapy with the proper education and training. In large part, however, general dentistry consists of restorative procedures. When a patient presents with dental caries, a proper diagnosis is made utilizing both clinical and radiographic examination when possible. Next, the affected tooth or teeth are prepared using drills and hand instruments in order to remove all carious and defective tissue while protecting the pulp. It is also important to create an appropriate design for the desired restorative material while conserving as much healthy tooth structure as possible. Finally, the appropriate restorative material is placed in order to restore the tooth to proper form, function and esthetics.

Classification of Carious Lesions

As previously mentioned, caries is the process which results in cavitation. The first classification of tooth cavitation and preparation was developed in the late 1800's by Dr. Greene Vardiman Black, or G.V. Black, often considered the founder of modern dentistry. G.V. Black described six classes of lesions based on anatomical location which are still widely used today (Figure 5.1).

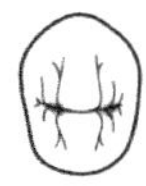

Class I lesions originate in pits and fissures of teeth, and are referred to as "pit-and-fissure lesions." Class I preparations occupy only one tooth surface, most commonly the occlusal surfaces of posterior teeth, lingual grooves of maxillary molars or buccal pits and grooves of mandibular molars.

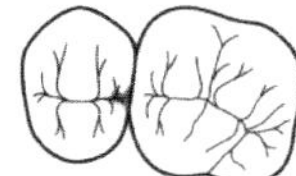

Class II lesions involve interproximal surfaces of posterior teeth. While Class II lesions may occupy only the proximal surface, preparations of these cavities include both proximal and occlusal surfaces

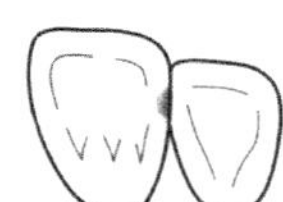

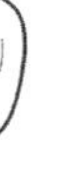

Class III lesions involve interproximal surfaces of anterior teeth but not their incisal edges.

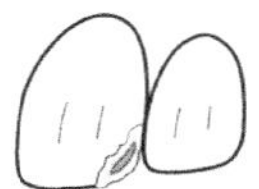

Class IV lesions involve both interproximal surfaces and incisal edges of anterior teeth. It should be noted that loss of an incisal edge is sometimes due to trauma rather than carious lesions.

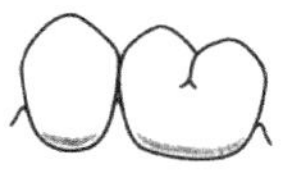

Class V lesions are located along the gingival margins of any tooth. Gingival margins act as plaque retentive areas where plaque may accumulate, causing white-spot lesions which progress to cavitated Class V lesions.

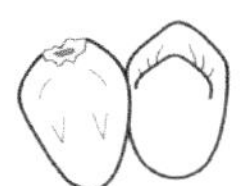

Class VI lesions involve cusp tips of canines, premolars and molars.

Figure 5.1 G.V. Black's classification of carious lesions.

Isolation

A clean and dry operating field is necessary for most restorative dental procedures. The physical properties of most restorative materials rely on a clean and dry tooth preparation, especially those that adhere to enamel and dentin. This type of field control can be achieved in many ways, such as using a rubber dam, gauze, cotton rolls, saliva ejectors, lip retractors and various absorbent or hemostatic materials.

Most dental schools support the use of the rubber dam as the most effective form of isolation (Figure 5.2). In this technique, the patient is first properly and adequately anesthetized. When working on a posterior tooth, a clamp is placed on the tooth distal to the tooth to be prepared to stabilize the rubber dam and sometimes to retract gingival tissue for preparations along the gingival margin. Holes for teeth are then punched out on the rubber dam material, commonly a thin 6 x 6" latex sheet. The dam is stretched over the selected teeth and held in position with a frame. Finally, floss is passed through the contacts to ensure complete adaptation of the rubber dam.

The advantages of the rubber dam are indisputable. The rubber dam improves operatory efficiency by allowing both improved access and visibility for the dentist as well as easier debris containment and water evacuation for the dental assistant. The rubber dam also protects the patient from swallowing or inhaling any debris from the preparation or restorative materials. As mentioned, physical properties of restorative materials are optimized in a clean and dry environment. The rubber dam does, however, take some time and practice for proper application. While dentists who decide to use rubber dams usually delegate the task to their assistants, dental students have to place the rubber dam themselves for many operative procedures. Despite time lost for placement, the improved operating efficiency and optimal material properties gained from the rubber dam maintain its use in dentistry.

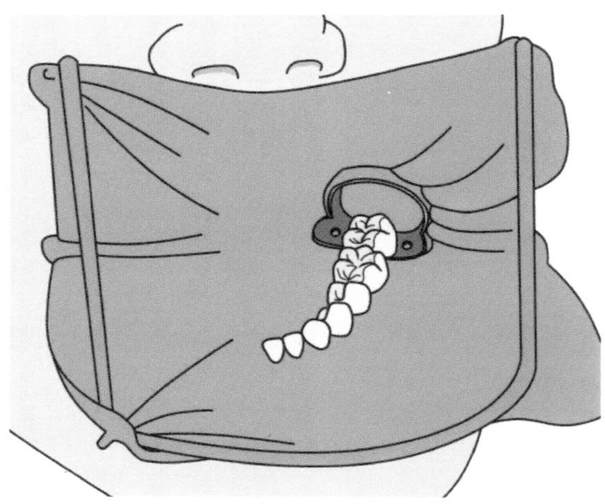

Figure 5.2 The rubber dam is the gold standard for isolation in dentistry.

Principles of Tooth Preparation

When Dr. G.V. Black first defined the principles of tooth preparation, he did so with one underlying principle in mind: "extension for prevention." This principle implied that a dentist may assume that a small lesion will eventually develop into a larger lesion, and the dentist was to extend the preparation into healthy tooth structure as a preventive measure. However, the indication for extension today is relatively minimal due to more effective prevention and treatment of caries, and is now based almost exclusively on the presence of caries and the restorative material to be placed. For example, a composite restoration can be placed in a more conservative tooth preparation than an amalgam restoration, for reasons discussed in the "Direct Restorations" section. The principles originally outlined by G.V. Black, however, are still in use today as follows:

Convenience form Obtaining convenience form refers to gaining sufficient access to the lesion to allow the dentist adequate visibility and instrumentation (Figure 5.3a,b). Usually this means making a "punch cut" with a high-speed drill and opening up the lesion enough to allow access with other burs used for caries removal.

Removal of carious dentin Caries extending beyond the enamel is usually removed with the largest round bur that will fit into the access created by convenience form using a slow-speed drill (6.5c). Because carious dentin is soft and demineralized, a slow-speed hand piece allows the dentist more tactile sensitivity to remove only the affected dentin. Hand instruments such as a spoon excavator can also be used to "scoop out" and scrape away carious dentin.

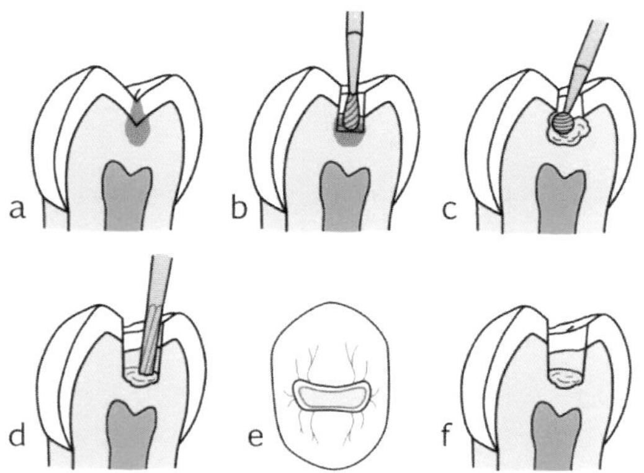

Figure 5.3 Sequence of caries removal and tooth preparation. First convenience form is achieved (b) followed by caries removal (c) and elimination of undermined enamel (d). Outline form is achieved in order to create a smooth margin (e). If additional retention is not indicated, the preparation may be cleansed (f) and assessed for restoration.

Removal of undermined enamel Any "overhanging" enamel is considered structurally undermined or compromised and should be removed with a high-speed drill (5.3d).

Outline form After removing caries and any undermined enamel, the outline and margins of the preparation may need to be modified so that they follow a gentle, free-flowing curve without sharp angles or jagged edges (5.3e). This optimizes the integrity of the margins at the junction of the tooth and the restoration.

Resistance form Resistance form refers to designing the cavity preparation in ways that prevent dislodgement of the restoration with angular forces or fracture during function. This can be achieved in several ways, including proper wall angulation, choosing an appropriate restorative material and adequate preparation depth to allow enough bulk of material to resist fracture.

Retention form This principle refers to the mechanical features of the preparation that keep the restoration in place and prevents dislodging it along the path of insertion, for example when chewing sticky foods that pull on the restoration. Retentive features include wall friction, internal grooves, points and pins. Retention and resistance forms are more important for restorative materials that do not bond or adhere to enamel or dentin, such as amalgam, as discussed in the "Direct Restorations" section of this chapter.

Cleanse the preparation The final preparation should be free from debris, rinsed out and dried for inspection and restorative material placement (5.3e).

Direct Restorations

Direct restorations are those which can be placed in one dental visit. A tooth is first prepared and the restorative material is immediately placed in the preparation by the dentist during the same appointment.

Composite

Composite is a tooth-colored material composed of acrylic resin and glass-like filler particles. Composite is the most commonly used restorative material for fillings and broken or chipped teeth, as well as inlays and veneers (discussed as indirect restorations). It may be either self-curing or light-cured with an intense blue light. Most light-cured composites are laid down in approximately 2mm-thick increments to allow adequate light penetration and curing efficiency.

The primary advantage of composite resin is the ability to accurately match tooth color and shade (Figure 5.4). Although not as strong as amalgam, current composites are comparable in strength and provide adequate reliability for small to mid-sized restorations withstanding moderate occlusal forces.

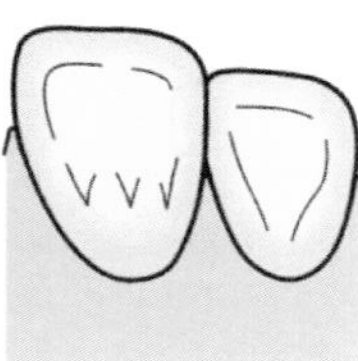

Figure 5.4 Composite restorations offer excellent color matching capabilities and adhesion to tooth structure.

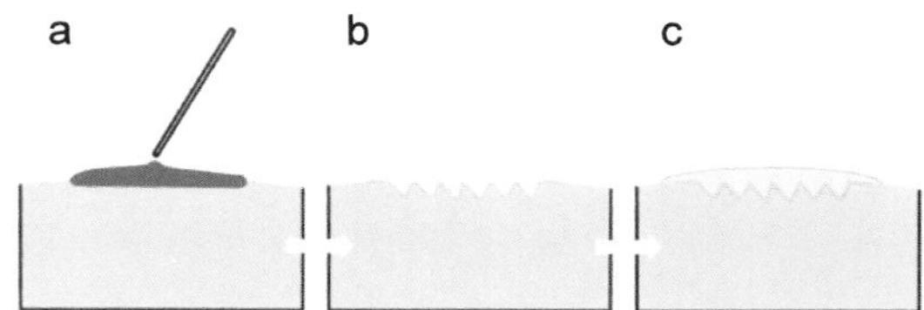

Figure 5.5 Adhesive systems utilize acid to incorporate microscopic irregularities on the surface of the tooth (a). The acid is rinsed and a primer is placed if dentin is exposed (b), followed by adhesive (c).

Another key feature of composite resins is their ability to bond to tooth structure using an adhesive system. While several different adhesive systems are available, the total-etch 3-step system is described. Cavity preparations are first etched with acid, usually a 37% phosphoric acid solution, in order to condition the preparation and selectively demineralize between 10 to 25 microns of the tooth surface, which selectively creates irregularities. Next, the acid etch is rinsed off and a primer is applied, which is only necessary when dentin is exposed. The final step in bonding, whether or not dentin is exposed, is placing an adhesive resin material to mechanically penetrate the irregularities created by the etchant, known as "resin tags" and chemically bond to the composite resin (Figure 5.5). Thus composite resins exhibit an effective micromechanical adhesion to tooth structure, eliminating the need to place additional retentive features into healthy tooth structure.

Disadvantages of composite resins include their susceptibility to moisture contamination during placement and polymerization shrinkage. Placing a composite restoration requires complete field control and a dry environment to prevent compromising both mechanical and adhesive properties. Furthermore, composite restorations are technique sensitive due to a small amount of shrinkage that occurs during the setting or polymerization reaction when the material is cured. The effects of polymerization shrinkage are minimized in the hands of a skilled dentist.

Amalgam

"Dental amalgam" refers to a mixture of approximately 43-54% mercury by weight with other metals, usually silver, tin and copper. The use of dental amalgam is constantly debated, however no public agency has definitively refuted the safety of dental amalgam fillings. Although toxic in its elemental form, mercury in dental amalgam is much more stable and less toxic than for example methylmercury, found in large fish such as tuna. Extremely small amounts of mercury vapor may be released from dental amalgam, however these are clinically insignificant amounts that are absorbed well below safety limits set by the federal government. Organizations such as the U.S. Food and Drug Administration (FDA) and the World Health Organization (WHO) concur on its general safety, and dental amalgams remain one of the oldest and most researched dental materials to date.[1,2]

There are several advantages to dental amalgam which maintain its use in dentistry. Amalgam can withstand relatively strong occlusal forces and is thus preferred for moderately-sized restorations in posterior teeth. It is also one of the only materials that is relatively unaffected by moisture and can be placed with a moist environment, which is particularly helpful for children or special needs patients when proper field control may be difficult. Amalgam exhibits minimal, if any, setting shrinkage and is self-sealing with resistance to further decay. Used for over 150 years in dentistry, amalgam is also generally the least expensive restorative material.

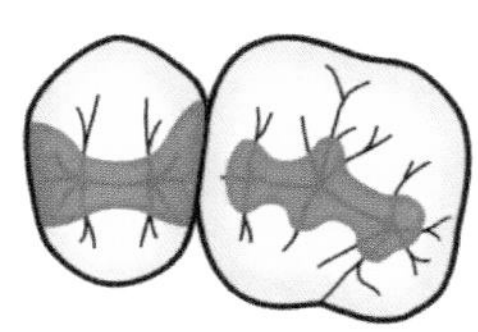

Figure 5.6 Amalgam restorations are generally reserved for moderate-sized restorations in posterior teeth.

The main disadvantage of amalgam is esthetics, another reason it is mainly reserved for posterior teeth (Figure 5.6). Amalgam also exhibits no adhesive properties and thus retentive features must be created within the cavity preparation, sometimes in the form of grooves or pins, which requires removing some healthy tooth structure. Given its mercury content, amalgam scrap left over from a restoration must be disposed of properly and requires special handling in order to protect the environment.

---

1 U.S. Food and Drug Administration (FDA), Consumer Update: Dental Amalgams, December 31, 2002.

2 World Health Organization (WHO), WHO Consensus Statement on Dental Amalgam, September, 1997.

Conventional Glass Ionomer

Conventional glass ionomers are another option for a tooth-colored restorative material. They are composed of ion-leachable glass particles and polymerizable acids. Compared to composite or amalgam materials, glass ionomer is not as strong and thus mainly used for smaller restorations in areas that are not subject to heavy biting forces, especially useful for lesions on the root surfaces of teeth (Figure 5.7).

The primary advantage of glass ionomer is its ability to release fluoride and prevent further decay or even locally remineralize affected tooth structure, particularly useful for patients with poor oral hygiene. The fluoro-alumino-silicate glass particles actually release small amounts of fluoride and have even been shown to "re-charge" when exposed topically to fluoride in the oral environment. Esthetics may also be an advantage. Furthermore, tooth preparations for glass ionomer may be more conservative than for those of amalgam restorations.

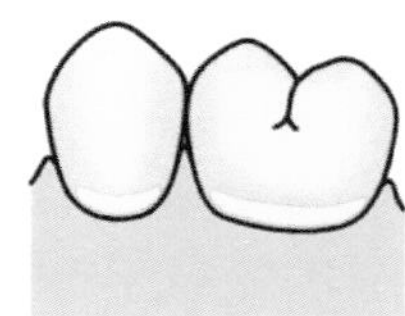

Figure 5.7 Glass ionomers release fluoride ions that protect the tooth well after placement.

As mentioned, conventional glass ionomers do not provide much resistance to fracture and are limited in their use to small restorations on non-occlusal tooth surfaces. Over time, this material can become susceptible to acidic environments and its surface may become rough or etched to harbor plaque. While conventional glass ionomers exhibit minimal polymerization shrinkage, the strength of their bond to tooth structure is less than that of composite resins. Cost may also need to be taken into consideration, as it is comparable to composite resins and more expensive than amalgam.

Resin-modified Glass Ionomer

A resin-modified glass ionomer (RMGI) is what its name implies - they are made from the same glass particles as conventional ionomers but have added acrylic resins for improved strength and decreased sensitivity to moisture. Although they are slightly stronger than conventional glass ionomers, RMGI's are still generally reserved for restorations with minimal biting forces in the adult dentition but can be more useful for short-term placement in primary teeth. As with conventional glass ionomers and composite resins, RMGI's can match tooth color and be placed in more conservative preparations than amalgam. However, they too are more expensive than amalgam and still exhibit some polymerization shrinkage.

Indirect Restorations

Indirect restorations require two or more dental visits. The dentist first prepares a tooth or several teeth and makes an impression of the area to be restored. This impression is then sent to a dental laboratory with detailed written instructions for the type of restoration the dentist would like to have fabricated. While the laboratory makes the permanent restoration, the dentist places an interim restoration in the preparation during the first appointment. Upon delivery of the permanent restoration, the dentist evaluates the restoration and cements it into place at the second appointment, making final adjustments as necessary. Indirect restorations include inlays, onlays, veneers, crowns and bridges. Materials used for indirect restorations include gold, porcelain ceramics and composite.

Inlays and Onlays

Inlays are intracoronal restorations, meaning they are contained within the occlusal tables of posterior teeth and do not cover cusps. For example, Class II lesions may be restored with an inlay (Figure 5.8a). Onlays are extracoronal restorations which cover one or more cusps (5.8b). Onlays may be indicated when there is an extensive loss of tooth structure, such as cracked teeth due to trauma. Endodontically treated teeth may also be good candidates for onlays.

Inlays and onlays are generally placed only on posterior teeth. Preparations for both inlays and onlays tend to be less conservative than their direct restoration counterparts. They also tend to be more technique sensitive, requiring much more precise drilling and strict adherence to preparation principles. The most popular materials for inlays and onlays are porcelain ceramics and gold. Due to the laboratory fee and expensive materials used, inlays and onlays are generally more expensive than direct restorations. However, with good oral hygiene habits these restorations can be incredibly durable and provide unmatched longevity.

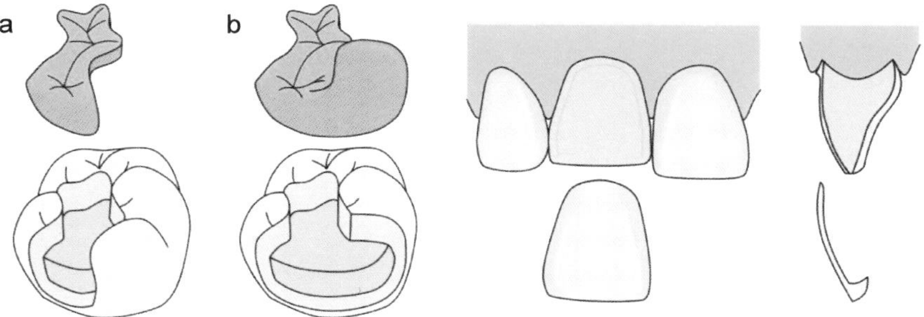

Figure 5.8 Inlays (a) and onlays (b) are commonly made from either gold or porcelain.

Figure 5.9 Veneers are used to correct a number esthetic of features on anterior teeth.

Veneers

Veneers are thin, custom overlays that cover the facial surfaces of teeth and are made from tooth-colored materials such as composites or porcelain (Figure 5.9). Veneers can treat diastemas (open spaces between teeth), chipped or intrinsically stained teeth, or even help reshape poorly shaped or crooked teeth. These restorations are permanent and irreversible, since a thin layer of enamel must be taken off to place and cement them, and they are usually indirect restorations made by a dental technician in the laboratory based on an impression made by the dentist.

Porcelain, although quite strong on compression, is weak on tension and thus may crack or chip due to its brittle nature and inability to flex. The dentist will also educate the patient to avoid certain foods that can stain veneers like coffee, dark soda and red wine.

Crowns and Bridges

Crowns and bridges are considered prosthodontic treatments and are discussed in the next chapter, Prosthodontics.

6

PROSTHODONTICS

Prosthodontics ("pros" for short) pertains to the diagnosis and treatment of patients with missing or deficient hard and soft tissues with prosthetic replacements. Natural teeth can be deficient due to trauma, caries or may be congenitally missing since birth. The role of a prosthodontist is to diagnose and restore deficient oral tissues to proper function and esthetics using biocompatible prosthetic materials. As specialists, prosthodontists tend to treat more difficult cases with complex treatment plans and may restore more implants than a general practitioner. Prosthodontic treatment, however, is not limited to prosthodontists. In fact general practitioners spend an estimated 20% of their time providing prosthodontic services to patients.[3]

Trends in prosthodontics show a bright future, with demand exceeding the current supply of prosthodontic treatment. The average number of teeth in a dentition decreases with age, falling from about 27 teeth in the average 18-24 year old to approximately 16 in persons 75 years of age or older.[4] Although life expectancy in the United States is increasing, and people are maintaining more of their natural teeth for longer periods of time, the elderly population continues to increase to offset the decrease in edentulism. While overall tooth retention in the United States is increasing, the increase in population size, in particular the elderly population, continues to increase the need for prosthodontic treatment. The elderly population of the Baby Boomer generation also have the means to finance their need for prosthodontic treatment. More information may be obtained about the specialty and career of prosthodontics from the American College of Prosthodontists (www.prosthodontics.org).

---

3 Nash KD, Douglass CW, Lipscomb J, Scheffler R, Wilson J. "Economies of scale and productivity in dental practices." Vol. 1, Final Report. Bureau of Health Manpower, Health Resources Administration, Department of Health and Human Services, Contract No. 231-75-0403. 1980.

4 Marcus et al., "Tooth retention and tooth loss in the permanent dentition of adults: United States, 1988-1991." Journal of Dental Research. 1996 Feb; 75 Spec No: 684-95.

Impressions and Casts

An impression is an imprint, or a "negative" of a dental arch and surrounding soft tissues used for the purpose of making a cast, or a "positive" model of a patient's dentition. Depending on the treatment, different types of impressions and casts can be made for diagnostic purposes and/or to aid in the fabrication of a definitive prosthesis.

During the initial prosthodontic appointment, a preliminary or "diagnostic" impression is made with a plastic or metal stock tray which comes in standardized sizes (Figure 6.1a). The impression material of choice is known as Alginate, a hydrocolloid material derived from seaweed. From this impression, a diagnostic cast made from gypsum stone is produced (6.1b). For some procedures, this cast may be adequate. For others, a custom impression tray must be fabricated in order to accomplish the most accurate anatomical reproduction possible.

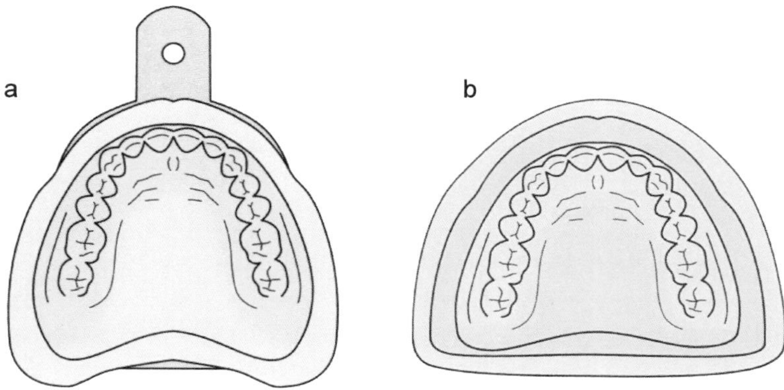

Figure 6.1 A diagnostic impression using a metal stock tray and alginate impression material (a) and a diagnostic cast poured in Type III gypsum stone, or "microstone" (b).

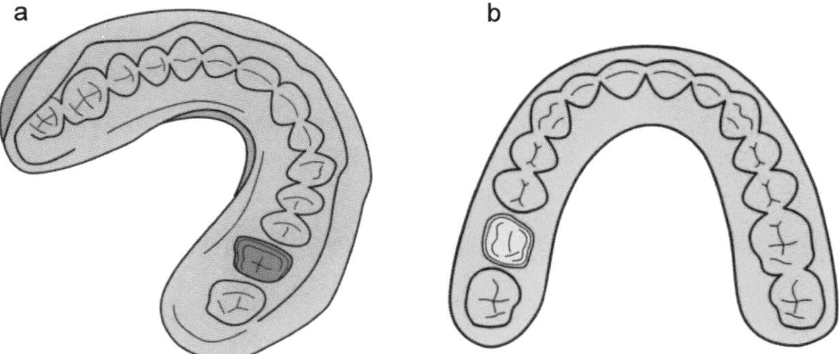

Figure 6.2 A master impression is created from Stern-Tek® custom tray material and PVS impression materials on the right (b). From the master impression, the master cast is poured in Type IV gypsum stone (b).

A custom impression tray is made by adapting an even thickness of wax to areas of the diagnostic cast to be included in the impression. A moldable tray material that can become rigid, such as Stern-Tek®, is then adapted around the wax and trimmed appropriately, leaving space for an even thickness of material around the teeth. From the custom impression tray, the master impression is made (Figure 6.2a). The same technique as for the diagnostic set is used, however this time utilizing the custom tray with a more accurate and dimensionally stable impression material, polyvinyl siloxane (PVS). The master impression is poured up with a type IV gypsum stone in order to produce the master or definitive cast (6.3b). The dental laboratory then uses this cast to fabricate a final prosthesis.

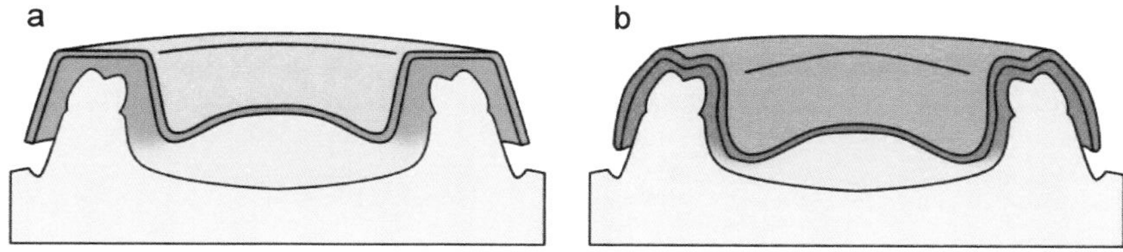

Figure 6.3 A stock tray only approximates the contours of the dentition (a) while a custom tray provides a precise and even layer of thickness between the teeth and the tray.

At first, the need for two different impressions and casts may not be clear. A stock tray will not fit evenly around the oral anatomy of every patient (Figure 6.3a). A custom tray is necessary because it follows the contours of one's dentition more precisely and the PVS material used with custom trays is most accurate at a thickness of 1 to 2 mm around the tooth preparation (6.3b).[5] The master casts that are made from these custom trays require very accurate anatomical reproduction in order to accurately reproduce the teeth and analyze how they occlude, or fit together. The prosthesis can then be fabricated based on this relationship. Digital impression techniques and technology, however, is becoming more prevalent in private practice and is slowly making its way into the dental school curriculum as well.

The Articulator

Master casts are mounted onto an articulator for the fabrication of a definitive prosthesis. An articulator is a device to which upper and lower casts are mounted in order to reproduce the positional relationships of a patient's upper and lower dentitions. Essentially, the purpose of the articulator in prosthodontics is to simulate the patient in their absence. The dentist can make several measurements of the patient's facial structure using a face bow (Figure 6.4a) and transfer this information to the articulator. Casts are used to simulate the patient's teeth and the condylar elements of the articulator simulate the patient's temporomandibular

---

[5] Nissan et al., "Effect of wash bulk on the accuracy of polyvinyl siloxane putty-wash impressions." Journal of Oral Rehabilitation. 2002 Apr; 29 (4): 357-61.

joints (6.4b). Using various settings on the articulator, a dentist or dental technician can then mimic the jaw movements of the patient and contour the definitive prosthesis according to the functional and anatomical needs of the patient.

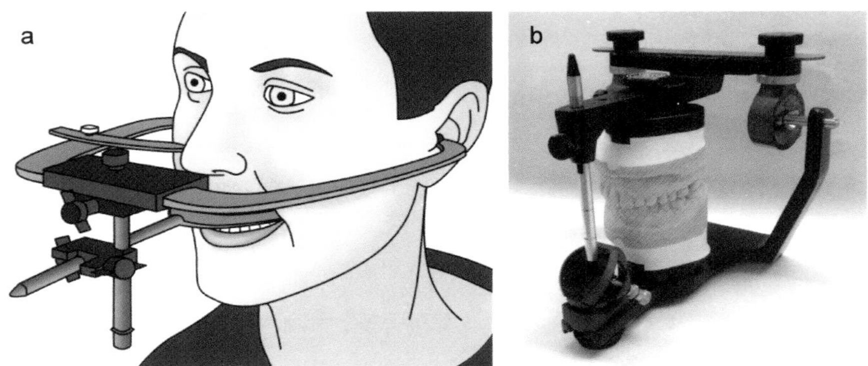

Figure 6.4 A facebow is used to relate the maxillary arch to the axis of the TMJ (a). A Hanau Wide-view articulator can be used to simulate the patient in order for the laboratory to fabricate a definitive restoration (b).

Fixed Prosthodontics

Fixed prosthodontics is the branch of prosthodontics which restores or replaces teeth using artificial substitutes that are cemented or otherwise fixed to teeth or implants. Those that are fixed to teeth include crowns and bridges, more formally known as fixed partial dentures. Crowns are single unit prostheses which restore single teeth whereas fixed partial dentures are usually attached to two or more teeth and replace missing teeth.

Crowns

A crown is a fixed restoration which covers most or the entire crown of a tooth. A crown may be considered in order to replace missing tooth structure, strengthen a weakened tooth or for esthetic reasons. Most crowns are made from porcelain, porcelain-fused to metal or metal.

When preparing a tooth for a crown, several biological, mechanical and esthetic principles must be kept in balance. A morphologic reduction preserves the basic anatomy of the tooth while conserving as much healthy tooth structure as possible; essentially the prepared tooth should look like a smaller version of itself. The master cast in Figure 6.2b exhibits a crown preparation for tooth #3. Retention and resistance form are key to the integrity and overall success of crowns and fixed prosthodontics in general. The opposing walls of the preparation must be close to parallel but also allow enough taper for the placement of the prosthesis. The contours of the crown itself must match that of the original tooth and when esthetics is a concern, must match harmoniously the surrounding teeth in color and shade.

Interim Restorations

With the exception of some all-ceramic (porcelain) crowns, which can be made in a single dental visit using CAD-CAM technology (computer-aided design, computer-aided manufacturing), crowns are fabricated by a dental laboratory, i.e. they are indirect restorations. After the tooth is prepared, the dentist makes an impression of the dentition and sends it to a dental laboratory. Meanwhile, the dentist must provide an interim or provisional restoration for the patient to wear while the definitive crown is being made (Figure 6.4). The interim restoration serves to protect the prepared tooth, maintain periodontal health and restores the tooth to function in mastication, phonetics and esthetics during this time. Interim restorations also maintain prepared teeth in their positions while definitive restorations are fabricated to avoid any drifting of the prepared tooth or adjacent teeth. In summary, the interim should serve the same purposes as a definitive restoration with the exception of longevity and less complex shade-matching.

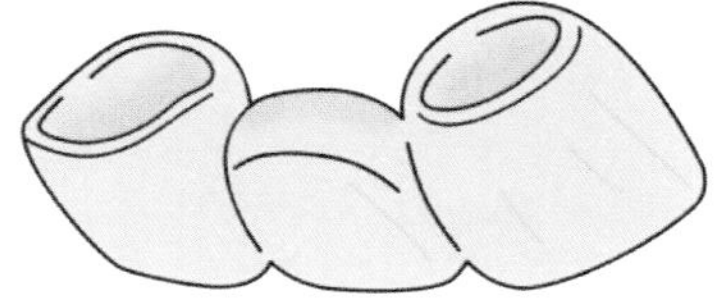

Figure 6.4 An interim restoration for a #6-8 bridge, or fixed partial denture, made from a poly methyl methacrylate (PMMA) material.

All-ceramic crowns (ACC)

Dental porcelain is a family of ceramic materials made of kaolin, quartz and feldspar which are fired at high temperatures. All-ceramic crowns may be fabricated either by a dental laboratory or a CAD-CAM system. The primary advantage of porcelain crowns is esthetics and the ability to most accurately match tooth color and translucency (Figure 6.5). Thus, all-ceramic crowns are particularly useful in the "esthetic zone" for anterior teeth. Their primary disadvantage is the intrinsic brittleness of porcelain materials. Because porcelain's strength depends on its thickness, all-ceramic crown preparations also tend to be less conservative and may require the removal of healthy tooth structure to allow for sufficient porcelain thickness of the crown.

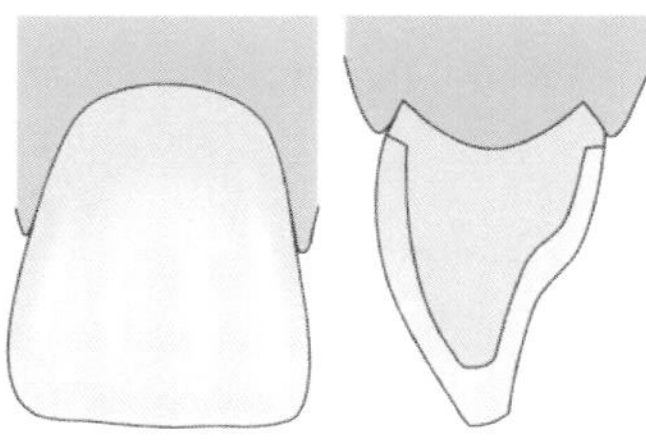

Figure 6.5 An all-ceramic crown provides optimum esthetics.

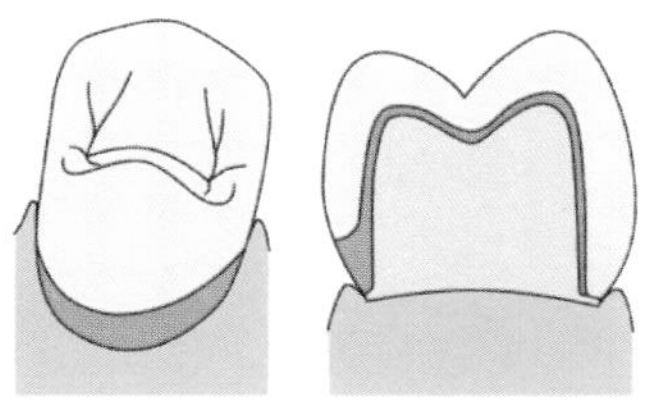

Figure 6.6 A porcelain-fused to metal crown contains a metal sub-structure which provide support for the overlying porcelain.

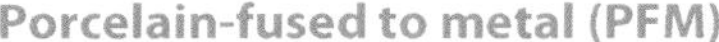

Porcelain-fused to metal (PFM)

Porcelain-fused to metal crowns consist of an outer porcelain layer which is fused to an underlying metal substructure (Figure 6.6). The metal substructure provides more strength and durability than all-porcelain crowns. PFM crowns also allow the dentist to mimic the appearance of natural teeth. However, translucency is limited by the metal substructure; i.e. a minimum thickness of porcelain is required in order to adequately mask the presence of metal. Thus PFM crowns may also be less conservative, requiring a porcelain thickness which balances optimal mechanical properties with esthetic goals.

Full-gold crowns (FCG)

Full-gold crowns are actually an alloy of gold, copper and other metals such as palladium (Figure 6.7). With a relatively higher strength in thin sections, preparations for gold crowns are more conservative than all-ceramic or porcelain-fused to metal crowns. Gold is also more gentle to natural teeth when compared to porcelain, which may wear or grind down opposing teeth. The primary disadvantage of full-gold crowns is poor esthetics, lacking the ability to mimic a natural tooth.

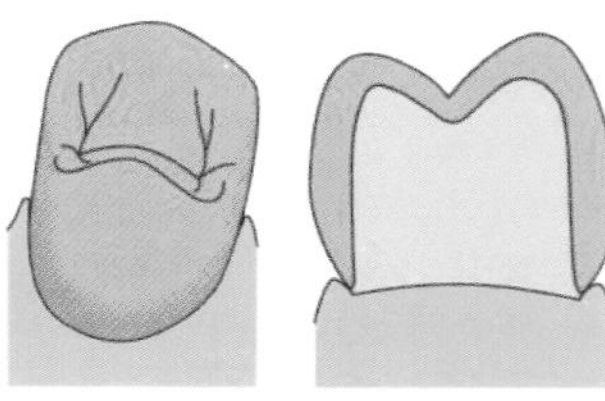

Figure 6.7 A full-gold crown provides the best strength and durability, and wears most similar to natural teeth.

Fixed Partial Dentures

A fixed partial denture (FPD), commonly known as a bridge, is a dental prosthesis which is cemented or otherwise fixed to at least two crowns, roots or implants for the purpose of replacing a missing tooth or several missing teeth. (Figure 6.8) The requirements for a fixed partial denture are similar to those of a crown, except that two or more teeth must be taken into consideration instead of just one. An impression of the preparation is sent to the dental laboratory, and an interim restoration must be provided by the dentist while the dental laboratory fabricates the final restoration utilizing casts mounted to an articulator. Some new terminology may also be helpful when referring to fixed partial dentures:

Abutment
Either a natural tooth or an implant which serves as the support and attachment of the fixed partial denture.

Retainer
The portion of the FPD which is cemented or other-wise secured to the abutment(s).

Pontic
The part of the restoration which is suspended from retainers which acts to replace the missing tooth or teeth.

Connector
The portion of the FPD which connects pontics to retainers.

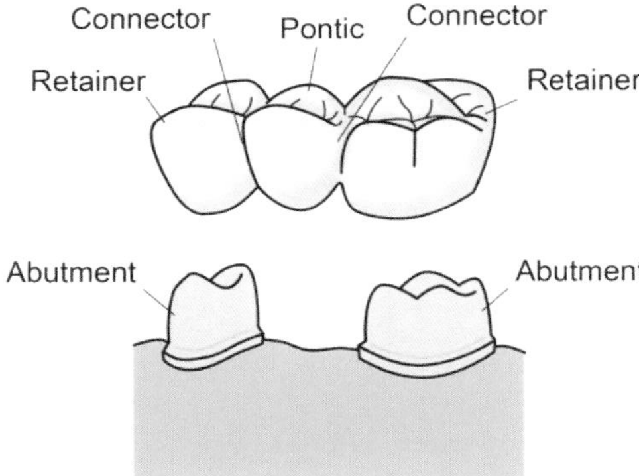

Figure 6.8 A typical 3-unit bridge replacing a single tooth, composed of two retainers cemented to abutment teeth connecting to a single pontic.

Removable Prosthodontics

Removable prosthodontics is the branch of prosthodontics which replaces teeth using devices which can be readily inserted and removed by the patient. These prosthetic appliances may be retained in the mouth by natural teeth, surrounding hard and soft tissues, implants and/or various combinations of these components. Complete dentures replace all teeth in a completely edentulous arch, i.e. one that is missing all teeth, whereas removable partial dentures (RPD's) replace teeth in a partially edentulous arch.

Complete Dentures

A complete denture is a removable appliance which replaces all the teeth and associated structures in one or both dental arches. A complete denture may be retained either by the remaining anatomical structures in the mouth or fixed to implants (discussed in Implant Prosthodontics).

When all teeth in either the maxillary or mandibular arch have been lost or extracted, they leave behind an edentulous ridge, which is simply the alveolar process and overlying gingiva which originally housed the teeth. In general, a maxillary denture is better retained in the mouth due to an increased surface area provided by the hard palate, while mandibular dentures are limited by the presence of the tongue and rely heavily on the edentulous ridges for retention. Regardless, edentulous ridges are dynamic structures which usually continuously decrease in size once teeth are lost. This is because when the bone of the alveolar process is not stimulated by the mechanical stress of functional teeth, the supporting bone tends to resorb or retract, which effectively decreases the amount of support available for dentures.

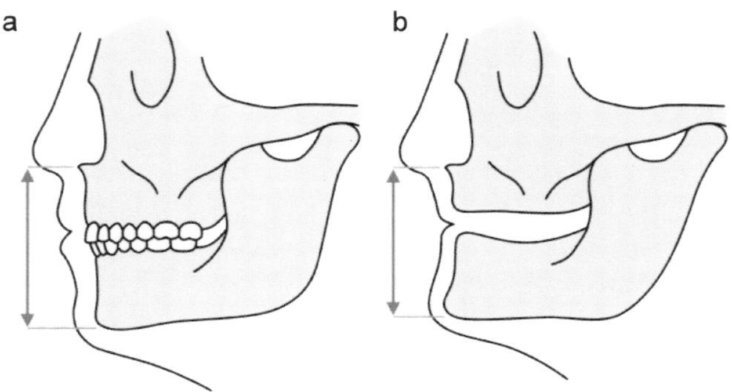

Figure 6.10 In a normal dentition, the lips are supported, the mandible is in a normal position and the vertical dimension of the face is maintained (a). Withou teeth, vertical dimension is decreased (b).

Like most prosthodontic services, complete dentures require several appointments. During the preliminary appointments, a treatment plan is discussed with the patient and diagnostic casts are produced, from which custom trays are made.

One feature almost exclusive to complete dentures is the need to determine a proper vertical dimension for the new prosthetic dentition. Teeth play a vital role in proper facial structure and support (Figure 6.10a). When absent, a patient's lips have the appearance of 'falling' into the mouth due to a lack of support from teeth and the mandible tends to rotate up and forward, in effect shrinking the face vertically (6.10b). Complete dentures reestablish lip support as well as the vertical dimension of the face.

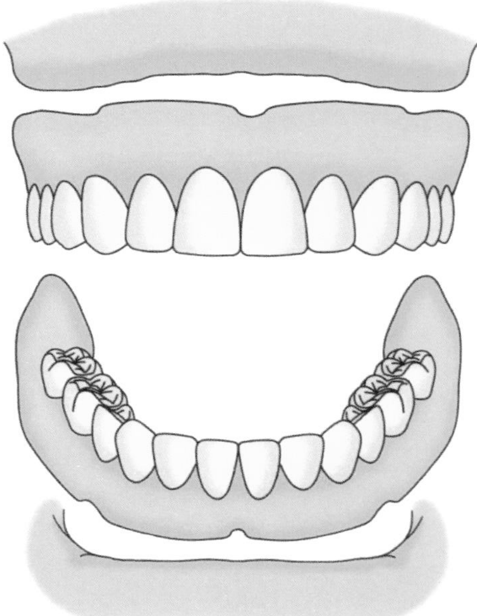

Figure 6.11 Complete upper and lower dentures replace all teeth in the edentulous arches.

Once proper positioning is determined, a wax denture is fabricated utilizing definitive casts mounted on an articulator. The wax denture is created by producing a wax occlusal rim to simulate the periodontium, into which denture teeth are set and articulated. This "trial" denture is then tried in the patient's mouth to verify proper esthetics and phonetics as well as proper occlusal relationships. If both the dentist and the patient approve, the wax dentures are sent to the laboratory for processing and fabrication of a definitive prosthesis.

During the delivery appointment, the complete dentures are presented to the patient and final adjustments are made (Figure 6.11). Post-operative appointments are also necessary to assess the dentures as well as the surrounding oral tissues. The patient must be made aware that the dentures may need to be relined or even replaced as hard and soft tissues change with time.

It is also important to note that as a dentist you have the freedom to choose how much of the process you take part in. For example, setting denture teeth in wax can be a tedious process which many dentists delegate to specialized technicians.

Removable Partial Dentures

A removable partial denture (RPD) offers an alternative to fixed partial dentures to replace teeth in a partially dentate arch. In a basic sense, a removable partial denture consists of a metal framework attached to an acrylic material into which denture teeth are set (Figure 6.12). However, the design components of each removable partial denture are individualized to each patient based on their remaining dentition. Removable partial dentures may be retained in the mouth by natural teeth, implants or a combination of the two with various clasps and other retentive features to help stabilize them.

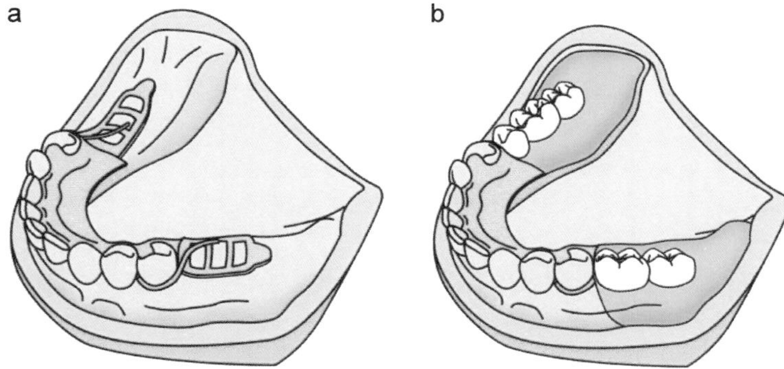

Figure 6.12 A metal framework is first fabricated using a definitive cast (a). Acrylic denture base and denture teeth are then added to the framework (b).

Although fixed prosthodontic appliances may be preferred by many dentists and patients under favorable circumstances, removable appliances may be the treatment of choice in some situations. For example, a fixed partial denture relies on the presence of at least two abutment teeth. When no distal abutment exists, or a relatively long edentulous span exists compared to available abutment teeth, removable partial dentures become a more favorable treatment option. Implants may also correct these problems, however due to economic constraints removable partial dentures may remain the treatment of choice for some patients. Another situation in which removable appliances may be desirable is when teeth have been missing for a prolonged period of time and the remaining ridge has resorbed considerably. A fixed appliance would require abnormally long pontic teeth or grafting surgery in order to rebuild the ridge. Because removable partial dentures possess an acrylic component overlaying and supplementing the ridges, prosthetic denture teeth may be set regardless of ridge resorption and improve esthetics.

Implant Prosthodontics

Implant prosthodontics is a relatively new branch of dentistry that is increasing in both success and popularity. A dental implant is a prosthetic device which is inserted directly into bone and provides a surgical means to replace both crown and root portions of missing teeth. They offer stability by fusing to bone in a process known as osseointegration. Candidates for implant surgery must, however, have healthy gingival tissues and proper bone volume and density in order for implant surgery to be successful. Bone grafts and sinus lift procedures may be indicated prior to implant placement.

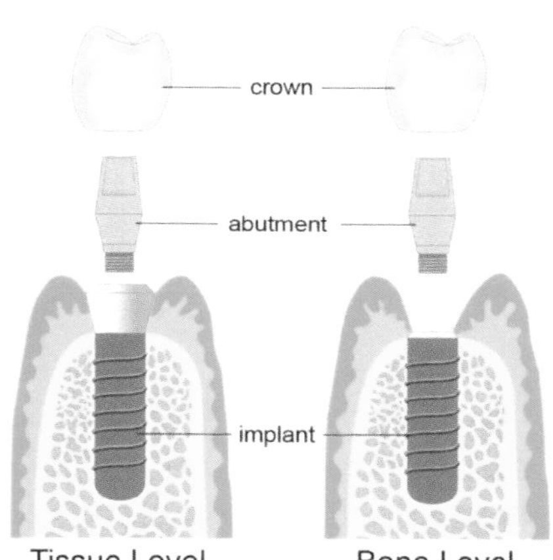

Figure 7.13 Dental implants consist of an implant, an abutment and the definitive restoration, such as a crown in the case of a single tooth implant. Implants may be set to either bone or tissue level.

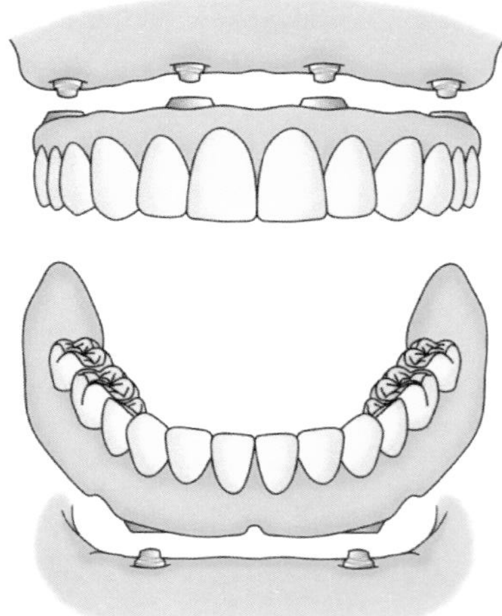

Figure 7.14 An implant-supported denture usually requires four to six implants (top), whereas an implant-retained denture usually suffices with two (bottom).

A dental implant consists of an implant, an abutment and the restoration, such as a crown in the case of a single tooth implant (Figure 7.13). The implant acts as the "anchor" which is inserted into bone and to which the abutment is secured. Implants may be either "tissue level", inserted to the level of the gingiva, or "bone level" and hidden under the gingiva to the height of the bone. An abutment is essentially a post which serves as a support and attachment apparatus, secured to the implant as well as the crown or other prosthesis.

In addition to replacing one or several missing teeth, dental implants may be placed to provide added support and/or retention for dentures (Figure 7.14). An implant-supported denture is one that relies completely on implants for support and usually requires four to six implants. Alternatively, an implant-retained denture is used if a patient's ridges support a complete denture but cannot retain it in a stable position. In this case, two implants may be placed posterior to the canine-premolar area to provide retention. The patient can then "snap" these dentures in and out of place, similar to a removable partial denture.

Maxillofacial Prosthetics

Prosthodontists may be involved with the prosthetic replacement of more than just teeth. Treatment including maxillofacial prosthetics is often coordinated with other medical and dental specialties. For example a prosthodontist may be asked to fabricate a prosthetic eye or an ear that was surgically removed due to cancer. Or perhaps one may be assigned to make an obturator, a device used to provide a barrier between the oral and nasal cavities in patients with a cleft palate. The fabrication of complex maxillofacial prosthetics may require supplementary training in addition to a prosthodontic residency program.

Reviewed by

Dr. James Clancy, D.D.S., M.S.
Associate Professor, Department of Prosthodontics
University of Iowa College of Dentistry

7

ORAL PATHOLOGY AND RADIOLOGY

Introduction to Oral Pathology

The specialty of oral pathology is the field of dentistry concerned with the diagnosis and treatment or management of diseases affecting the oral and maxillofacial regions. A proper diagnosis commonly includes a clinical and radiographic evaluation, as well as a microscopic or biochemical examination if needed. If a general dentist encounters a lesion with a potentially serious or complex diagnosis, a biopsy should be taken from a representative portion of the lesion and sent to an oral pathologist for evaluation. More information on the specialty can be found from the American Academy of Oral and Maxillofacial Pathology (www.aaomp.org).

Clinical Examination and Descriptive Terminology

After a detailed patient interview, which includes the history of the problem and pertinent medical and behavioral information, the dentist will examine the lesion or involved tissues and document the information into the patient's electronic health record. The location, size and distribution are noted, e.g. localized swelling of the posterior lateral border of the tongue measuring 6 mm in diameter and 2 mm thick. The shape, color and borders of the lesion are also important, e.g. a red-blue dome-shaped lesion with well-circumscribed borders. Palpation of the lesion provides information with regard to the surface contour and textures, and whether the lesion is freely movable or fixed to surrounding structures, a feature commonly exhibited by oral cancers.

From a medical and legal standpoint, it is important to document areas of concern in the most accurate and descriptive way possible. For example, when monitoring a lesion over a period of time, a thorough description allows for a precise comparison of features between dental visits. A brief review of common descriptive terms can be found in Table 7.1 and Figure 7.1.

Table 7.1 Common descriptive terms for oral lesions.

Term	Description
Macule	A flat area of color change
Papule	A solid, raised lesion less than 5 mm in diameter
Nodule	A solid, raised lesion greater than 5 mm in diameter
Vesicle	A fluid-filled blister less than 5 mm in diameter
Pustule	A fluid-filled blister with purulent discharge
Erythematous	Red in color
Leukoplakic	White in color
Edematous	Accumulation of excessive fluid in subcutaneous tissue
Exophytic	Growing outward
Endophytic	Growing inward
Ulcer	Loss of surface epithelium
Indurated	Abnormally hard
Sessile	Attached by a base, dome-shaped
Pedunculated	Attached by a stalk, narrower at its base
Papillary	Numerous surface projections
Verrucous	A rough, warty surface

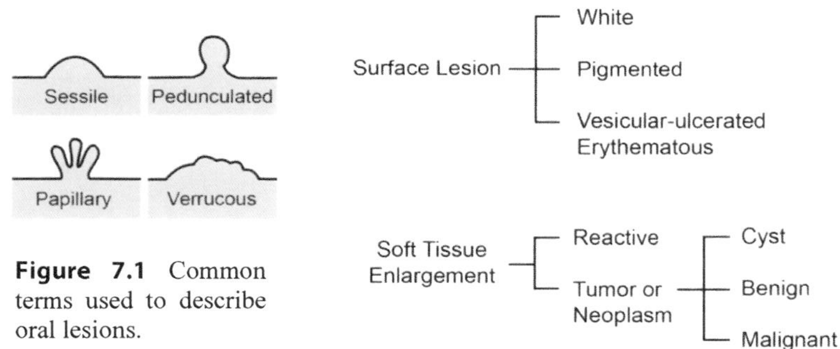

Figure 7.1 Common terms used to describe oral lesions.

Figure 7.2 A decision chart commonly used with soft tissue lesions of the oral mucosa.

Characteristics of Soft Tissue Lesions

Soft tissue lesions can be classified based on their site of origin. The first type, surface lesions, involve the epithelium only. Surface lesions are either flat or slightly raised, usually not exceeding 2-3 mm in thickness and often appear as either white, pigmented or ulcerated, vesicular and erythematous (red) in appearance. The second type, connective tissue lesions, arises either from the connective tissue itself, or the components contained within the connective tissue, i.e. blood vessels, salivary glands, or nerves. Connective tissue lesions generally do not alter the surface mucosa, though they may become ulcerated if they grow larger.

The first decision a dentist makes with a soft tissue lesion of the oral cavity is whether is it a surface lesion involving epithelium and superficial connective tissue or a soft tissue enlargement, commonly presenting as a mass or swelling. Surface lesions are either flat or slightly raised, usually not exceeding 2-3 mm in thickness and often appear as either white, pigmented or ulcerated, vesicular and erythematous (red) in appearance.

Soft tissue enlargements may either be reactive or tumorous/neoplastic. Reactive lesions are those caused by infection or injury, such as trauma or allergic reaction. These lesions have a rapid onset, are often symptomatic or painful and tend to fluctuate in size. A tumorous (tumor-like) lesion may either be a cyst (a fluid-filled sac) or a benign or malignant neoplasm (cancer). Soft tissue tumors are characterized by persistence and progression, in other words they do not resolve or fluctuate in size and in fact consistently increase in size. Tumors have a slow onset and tend to be asymptomatic but may present with systemic manifestations during late stages. Benign tumors tend to be well-circumscribed, freely movable and exhibit slow growth (months to years). Malignant neoplasms, on the other hand, tend to be infiltrative, poorly circumscribed and fixed to underlying structures. They also exhibit more rapid growth (weeks to months) and can be symptomatic or exhibit systemic manifestations. A sample decision process diagram is shown in Figure 7.2.

Introduction to Oral Radiology

Oral and maxillofacial radiologists are experts at interpreting oral and maxillofacial radiographs. This field of dentistry requires an intimate knowledge of normal and pathological anatomy in order to distinguish between the two. In addition to a clinical examination, radiographic images are one of the most important diagnostic tools available to a dentist, especially for hard tissue (bony) lesions. Although radiographs are limited in detail and portray three-dimensional objects in two dimensions, they provide useful information in areas that would otherwise require surgical intervention. More information may be obtained from the American Academy of Oral and Maxillofacial Radiology (www.aaomr.org).

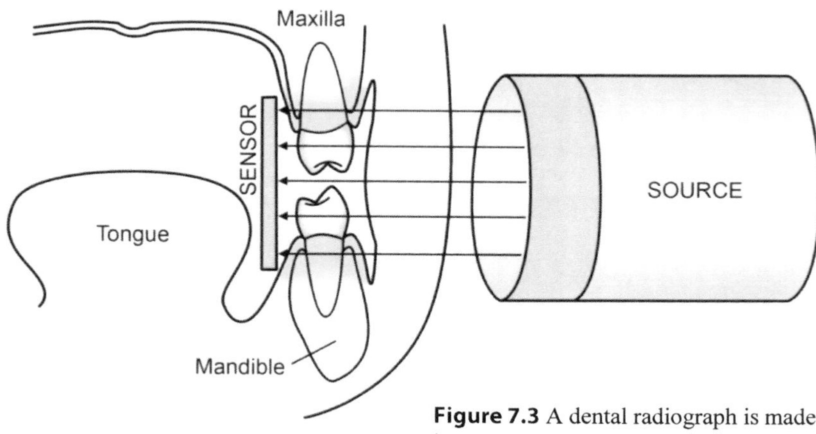

Figure 7.3 A dental radiograph is made by placing teeth between the sensor and the source of radiation.

Radiographic Imaging

In its most basic form, a radiograph is made by emitting x-rays from a source onto a sensor (Figure 7.3). Objects between the source and the sensor attenuate or block radiation at different intensities depending on their density. Thus, a radiograph is an image based on differences in densities. Dense substances block x-rays more than porous ones and are termed radiopaque, appearing white on a radiograph. Less dense or porous substances are termed radiolucent. They allow x-rays to pass through them more easily and appear grey or black on a radiograph.

Enamel is the most dense substance in the body, followed by dentin and then bone. Hence on a radiograph, enamel appears white, dentin light grey and bone a darker shade of grey.

Bitewing Radiographs

A bitewing (BW) radiograph is one that captures the crowns of upper and lower posterior teeth (Figure 7.4). Bitewings are routinely used to detect caries, especially interproximal caries which tend to be difficult to assess clinically. These radiographs are taken at right angles to the teeth in order to minimize distortion. Interproximal overlap is also minimized in order to "open" the contacts between teeth. Two bitewings are generally made for the posterior teeth, one to assess the premolars and one for the molars. As reviewed in Chapter 4, the caries process demineralizes tooth structure and presents as a radiolucency on a radiograph.

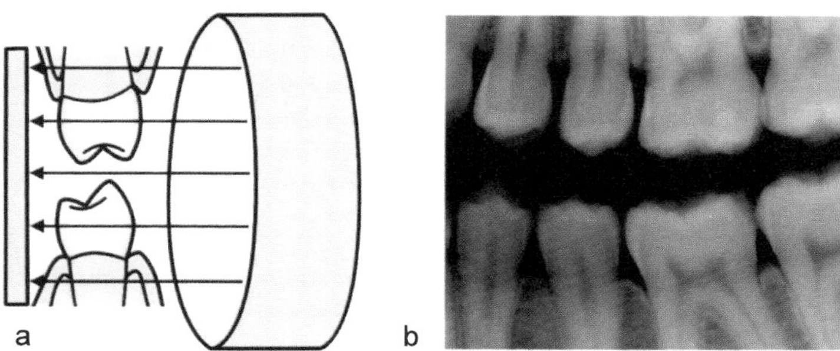

Figure 7.4 A bitewing radiograph captures the crowns of the upper and lower posterior teeth.

Periapical Radiographs

Periapical (PA) radiographs are made to assess the root and surrounding tissues of teeth, a region known as the periapex (Figure 7.5). These radiographs should capture the whole tooth as well as several millimeters below the root apex. Periapical radiographs are especially important in endodontics in order to evaluate the extent of an infection into the jaw bones as well as to assess healing after root canal therapy.

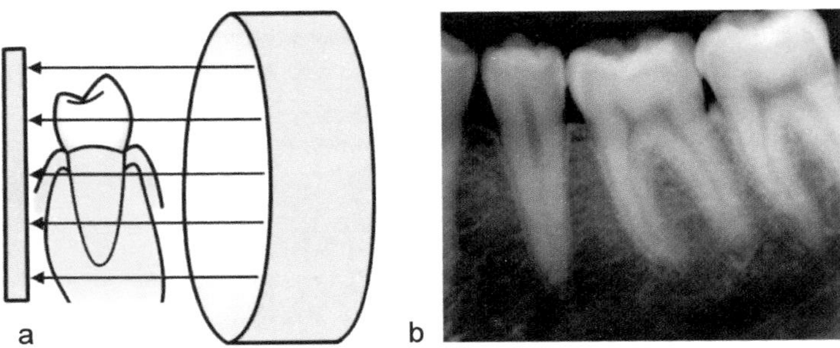

Figure 7.5 A periapical radiograph captures the whole tooth and bone around the root apex.

Complete Mouth Series

A complete mouth series, or CMS, is a series of twenty radiographs used to thoroughly evaluate the condition of the teeth and supporting bone. The CMS is a combination of bitewings and periapical radiographs of the all of the teeth (Figure 7.6).

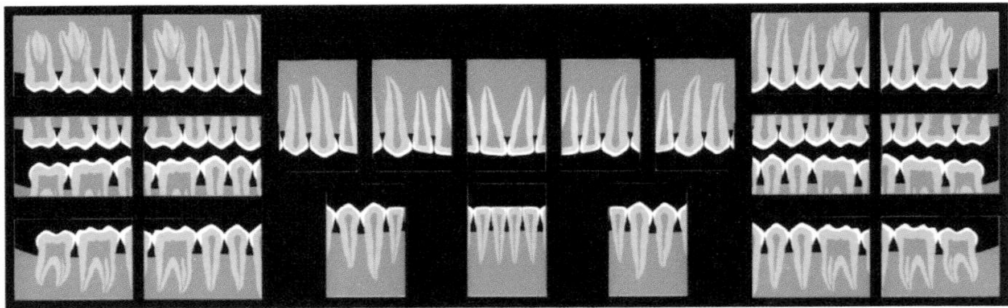

Figure 7.6 A complete mouth series (CMS).

Pantomographs

A pantomograph is a diagnostic tool which provides a panoramic view of the oral cavity and surrounding tissues (Figure 7.7). Pantomographs are useful in capturing large-scale information outside the limits of normal bitewing or periapical radiographs and is thus not used for diagnosing caries. Pantomographs are most commonly and routinely used to assess the anatomical position and development of third molars prior to their extraction as well as to visualize other areas such as the sinuses and temporomandibular joints.

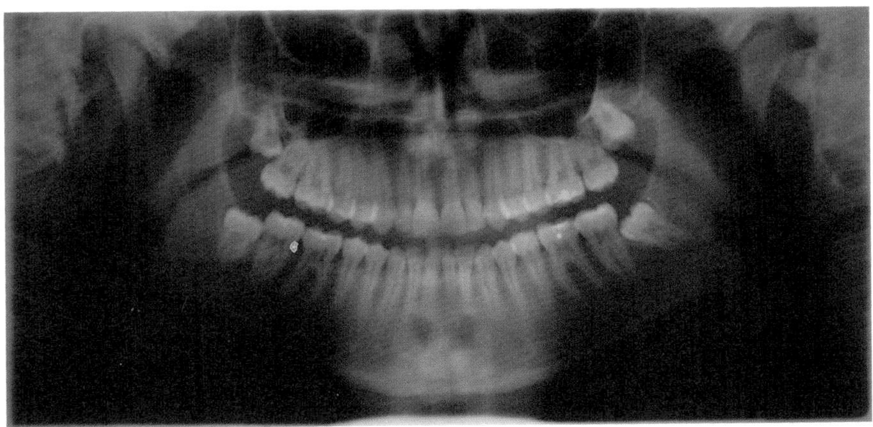

Figure 7.7 A pantomograph is a panoramic radiograph of the oral cavity and surrounding tissues.

Reviewed by
Dr. Ali Pourian, D.D.S., M.S.
Resident, Department of Oral and Maxillofacial Radiology
University of Iowa College of Dentistry

8

PEDIATRIC DENTISTRY AND ORTHODONTICS

Introduction to Pediatric Dentistry

Pediatric Dentistry ("pedo" for short) is widely known as an age-specific specialty that provides both preventive and comprehensive dental treatments for infants and children through adolescence, including those with special health care needs. The American Academy of Pediatric Dentistry (www.aapd.org) is the leader in representing the oral health interests of children and recommends that a child sees a dentist either by one year of age or when their first "baby" tooth erupts.

The Pediatric Patient

Children make pediatric dentistry a unique experience and add dimension to conventional practices. Aside from having smaller mouths and fewer teeth, kids are smaller in general and often require medication or anesthetic dosage modifications due to their smaller size and developing bodies. Pediatric dentistry can also be largely defined by behavior management. There are many philosophies on managing the behavior of the pediatric patient and with many children, a "tell, show, do" approach is sufficient. This refers to thorough explanation and demonstration with every procedure. Nitrous oxide (laughing gas) can be used to improve cooperation in children with moderate levels of anxiety. At times, when treatment is not urgent, it may be delayed due to a lack of cooperation. When treatment is urgent, and when nitrous oxide is inadequate, additional measures such as conscious sedation, medical immobilization (physical restraints) or general anesthesia may be required in order to provide the necessary treatment.

Pediatric dentists also treat many special needs patients, or those with a physical, developmental, mental, behavioral or cognitive condition that requires medical management, health care intervention or the use of specialized services or programs. Patient with special health care needs face additional challenges and barriers to receiving dental treatment and represent an underserved population which requires extra attention from pediatric and general dentists alike.

Primary Dentition

There are normally a total of 20 primary teeth. The primary dentition consists of 8 incisors, 4 canines and 8 molars (Figure 8.1). As is the case with permanent teeth, primary mandibular teeth tend to erupt before primary maxillary teeth. First to erupt are the primary mandibular central incisors, usually at about 6 months of age. After the rest of the incisors have erupted, a child's primary first molars, commonly referred to as "1st year" or "12 month" molars, will erupt before their canines. Canines are next to erupt at about 18 months followed by the second molars, or "2nd year" or "24 month" molars, at about 2 years of age. It may come to your attention that a primary dentition lacks premolars. In fact a child's primary molars are replaced by the permanent premolars, which is an important factor in proper tooth alignment and orthodontics.

In general, the sequence of eruption is considered to be more important than the times at which teeth erupt. It should be noted that the eruption times listed are averages and the "normal" range varies widely from child to child. However, if a contralateral tooth fails to erupt within about 6-12 months after its counterpart a radiograph may be indicated to investigate the potential for tooth impaction or even pathosis. For example if the mandibular right canine has erupted and the left mandibular canine has not shown clinical signs of eruption, a radiograph can be ordered.

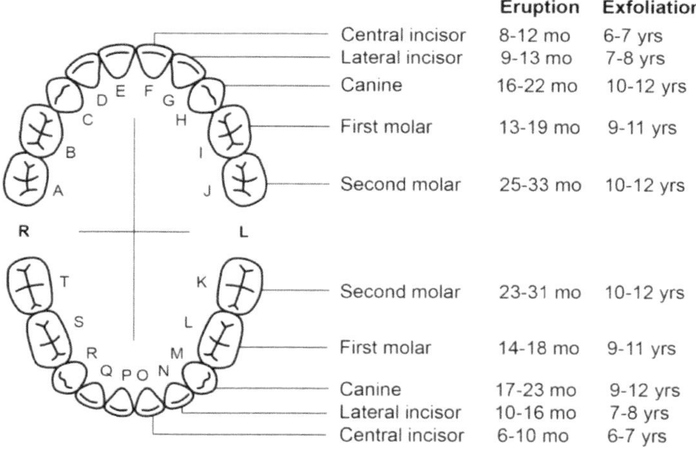

Figure 8.1 Eruption and exfoliation sequence of the primary dentition.

The most commonly used numbering system for primary teeth designates each one with a letter from A through T. The primary upper right second molar is deemed A, lettering from right to left until tooth J, the primary upper left second molar. Similar to the universal numbering system, deciduous numbering drops down to continue counting with the primary mandibular left second molar, K, and progresses through T, the primary mandibular right second molar. Although the primary system uses letters, many dentists will still refer to this as "numbering" teeth. This is because during pediatric dental appointments, many dentists tell children that they are looking inside their mouths to simply "count the teeth" in order to alleviate anxiety for the child.

Pediatric Restorations

In general the same restorative materials are used for children as are used for adults. However, glass ionomer and amalgam restorations may be used in a higher proportion due to their fluoride release and ease of placement, respectively. After caries removal, some of the design principles for primary teeth may differ as there are several differences between the primary and permanent dentition. For example, the pulp space is relatively larger in primary teeth than in permanent teeth (Figure 8.2). Thus moderate to large carious lesions may require pulp therapy and/or a stainless steel crown, described in the next section.

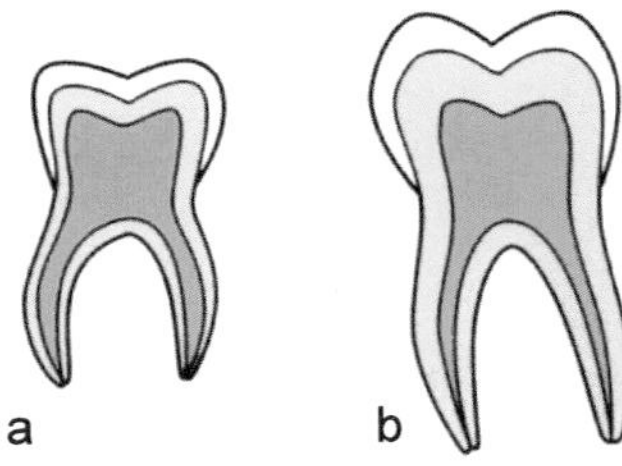

Figure 8.2 Although composed of the same tissues, morphology differs between primary (a) and permanent teeth (b).

Stainless Steel Crowns

First used in the 1940's, stainless steel crowns (SSCs) are primarily used in pediatric dentistry today. These crowns are very different from conventional gold or ceramic crowns used in the adult dentition. They are manufactured in standard sizes and can be considered a direct restoration since a laboratory is not needed in this process. The preparation for a stainless steel crown is also very different and more conservative than for a conventional crown. Stainless steel crowns are first tried in for size and then "crimped" around the edges with pliers for a more customized fit around the margins of the preparation. Once occlusion is verified the crown is cemented with a glass ionomer cement. Stainless steel crowns can be an economical and effective way to preserve the primary dentition (Figure 8.3).

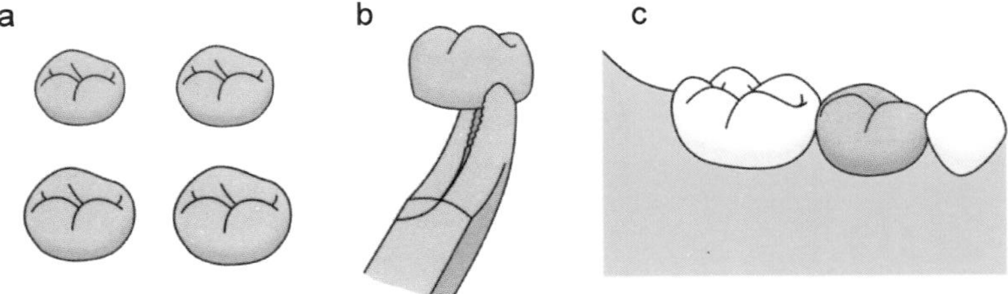

Figure 8.3 Stainless steel crowns (SSCs) are available in various sizes (a). The margins of the crown are "crimped" to fit the preparation (b) and the crown is cemented once occlusion is verified (c).

In general, stainless steel crowns are used for teeth with large carious lesions, as a permanent restoration following nerve treatments (pulpotemy or pulpectomy) and may even be attached to a space maintenance device if adjacent teeth are prematurely lost. For example, if a primary first molar is lost prematurely, a "crown and loop space maintainer" can be used to prevent mesial tipping or drifting of the primary second molar into the space where the permanent first premolar normally erupts. Essentially, a metal wire is attached to a stainless steel crown to retain the primary second molar in its position away from the primary canine in order to maintain that space (Figure 8.4).

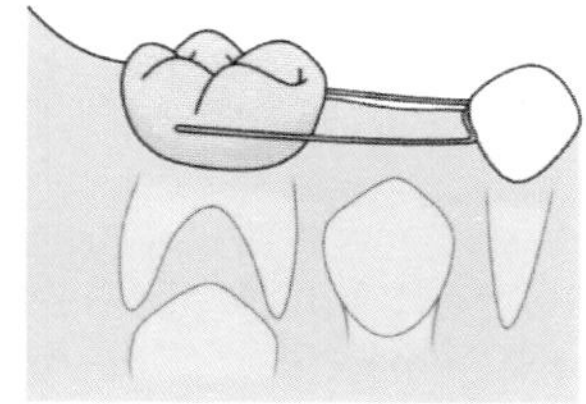

Figure 8.4 A crown and loop spacer may be indicated to maintain space in the arch for eruption of a permanent tooth.

Introduction to Orthodontics

Orthodontics is the dental specialty that may prevent, intercept and correct abnormal or irregular tooth position. As mentioned in Chapter 3, permanent teeth begin to erupt around age 6, at which point the dentition is known as a mixed or transitional dentition until all the primary teeth have exfoliated, usually around age 12. The American Association of Orthodontics (www.mylifemysmile.org) recommends that all children have an orthodontic check-up no later than age 7, with most orthodontic treatment beginning between the ages of 9 and 14.

When permanent teeth develop within the jaw bones, they can be visualized on a radiograph to aid in a complete analysis. This allows one to measure the length of the upper and lower arches as well as the total width of the teeth in each arch, i.e. to compare the space required by the teeth with the space available in the arch. If a general dentist decides that a child requires orthodontic therapy, he or she may be referred to an orthodontist in order to decide what treatment would be most appropriate. And although orthodontics is commonly started in children and adolescents, healthy teeth are moved in adults with the same orthodontic forces as those used in children.

Dentition Analysis and Evaluation

A thorough analysis of the dentition commonly includes both clinical and radiographic evaluations. Some common components to an analysis are reviewed.

Occlusion

Occlusion refers to how teeth bite together and function. A malocclusion refers to a "bad bite". It is not always easy to spot a malocclusion and many factors may contribute to a malocclusion. Some clues that may indicate the need for orthodontic attention include early or late loss of primary teeth, difficulty chewing or biting, crowded teeth, misplaced teeth or certain habits such as thumb-sucking, to name a few.

Several classes of occlusion exist, and the relationship of the canines and first molars are most commonly used to classify occlusion. Class I occlusion is the most favorable relationship of the teeth and jaws, where the cusp tip of the maxillary canine lies in between the mandibular canine and first premolar while the mesiobuccal cusp tip of the maxillary first molar lies in the buccal groove of the mandibular first molar. In a Class II relationship, the mandible is retruded from the Class I position while in a Class III relationship the mandible protrudes forward from Class I (Figure 8.5).

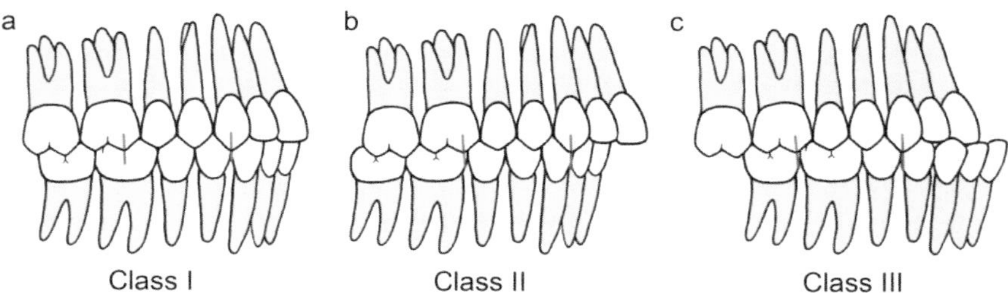

Figure 8.5 Class I is considered "normal" occlusion (a) while the mandibular arch is relatively retruded in Class II (b) or protruded in Class III occlusion (c).

Overbite vs. Overjet

Overbite and overjet are commonly mistaken terms. An overbite refers to the amount of overlap of anterior teeth in the vertical dimension, usually measured as a percentage of the mandibular anterior teeth. Overjet refers to overlap of the teeth in the horizontal direction, measured in millimeters from the facial surface of the maxillary anterior teeth to the facial surface of the mandibular anteriors (Figure 8.6).

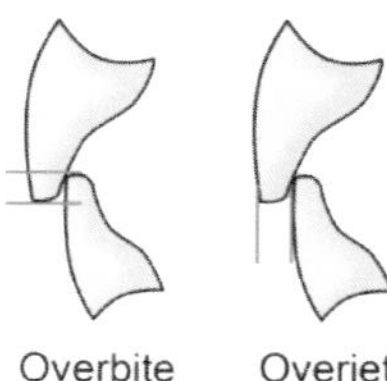

Figure 8.6 Overbite and overjet refer to vertical and horizontal overlap, respectively.

Anterior Open Bite

An anterior open bite occurs when an open space exists between the upper and lower anterior teeth while the posterior teeth occlude (Figure 8.7). Anterior open bites commonly result from oral habits such as thumb sucking or prolonged use of a pacifier. Once the oral habit is identified and eliminated, anterior open bites tend to correct themselves.

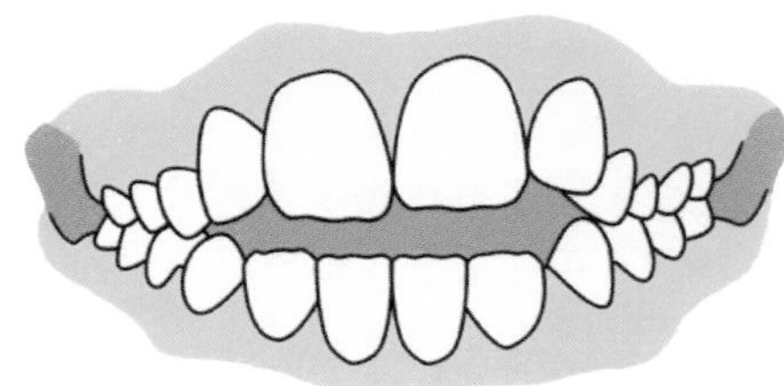

Figure 8.7 Anterior open bites commonly occur due to oral habits and tend to self-correct once the habit is controlled.

Anterior and Posterior Crossbites

In normal Class I occlusion, the maxillary anterior teeth overlap the mandibular anteriors in both the horizontal and vertical dimension. An anterior crossbite occurs if the maxillary anteriors tuck in under the mandibular anteriors, common in Class III occlusion. Posterior teeth normally occlude with the maxillary lingual cusps and the mandibular buccal cusps in their counterpart's central groove. A posterior crossbite may occur when the maxillary buccal cusps fall within the groove of mandibular teeth or when maxillary teeth are displaced completely lingual to mandibular teeth (Figure 8.8).

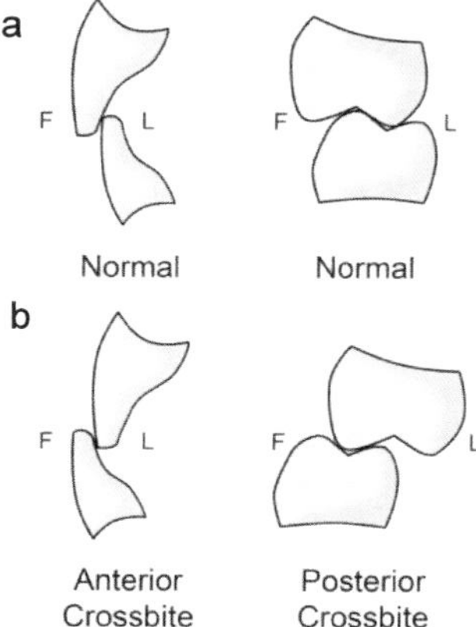

Figure 8.8 Compared to normal occlusion (a), the mandibular anterior teeth overlap maxillary anteriors and the facial cusp of maxillary posterior teeth occlude in the central groove of mandibular posterior teeth (b).

Spacing and Crowding

Spacing and crowding are common in the human dentition but may cause both esthetic and functional problems. Space between teeth, known as a diastema, may be inherent if teeth are too small for their dental arch or may develop as a consequence of a tooth extraction as teeth around the area shift to fill the void (Figure 8.9a). If diastemas are large enough, they may allow for adequate cleansing between teeth. Small diastemas, however, act as food traps and tend to wedge food between teeth. Crowding may also occur as a discrepancy between tooth size and room available in the dental arch, or may develop over time (8.9b). The tendency for teeth to shift toward the midline is known as "mesial drift", and may result in crowding. Crowding also results in difficult anatomy to properly cleanse with a brush and may present an increased caries risk.

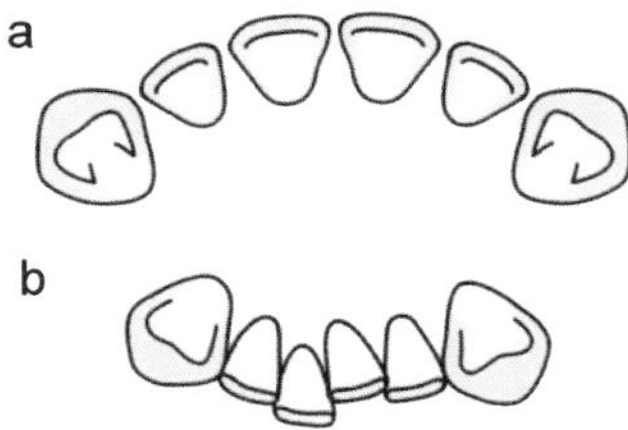

Figure 8.9 Diastemas may occur when teeth are too small for an arch or the arch is too large for the dentition (a) while crowding can result if the arch is insufficient or if the teeth are too large for the arch space (b).

Fixed vs. Removable Appliances

In general, fixed appliances, i.e. braces, are used when occlusion is complex or when the desired tooth movement requires control and precision. For example, tooth rotations and diastema closures are most effectively achieved with fixed orthodontic appliances. In Figure 8.10, a device known as a "2x4" (two by four) is shown in which two bands are placed around the permanent maxillary first molars for anchorage and connected to brackets on the four incisors via an orthodontic wire.

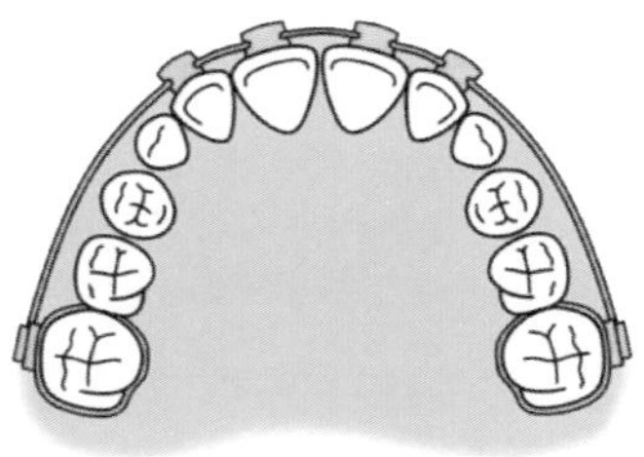

Figure 8.10 A "2x4" appliance can be used to rotate or straighten teeth with bands and brackets.

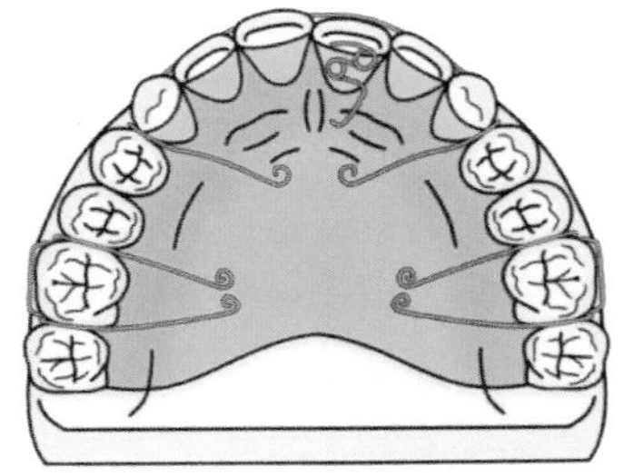

Figure 8.11 A removable Hawley appliance with a double-helix spring to tip tooth #9 facially.

Removable appliances are effective for more simple movements, such as tipping movements where space is available in the arch and occlusal clearance is adequate. For example, a removable Hawley appliance such as the one shown in Figure 8.11 can be utilized in order to move a single tooth facially. An impression is made of the arch and the cast is sent to a dental laboratory. The technician then fabricates a base using orthodontic resin and clasps to secure the appliance. Various springs or elastics can be incorporated into the appliance and "activated" to move teeth up to several millimeters. When the desired position is achieved, the springs are "deactivated" and the device is worn for a period of time in order to maintain its position in the arch.

Reviewed by

Dr. Michael Kanellis, D.D.S., M.S.
Professor, Department of Pediatric Dentistry
University of Iowa College of Dentistry

9

PERIODONTICS

Periodontics ("perio" for short) is the field of dentistry dealing with the diagnosis, treatment and prevention of diseases of the supporting tissues of the teeth (the periodontium). Although periodontal treatment may be limited to scaling and root planing for some patients, periodontics is a surgical specialty which also provides dental implant placement. The American Academy of Periodontology represents the specialty of periodontics and more information can be found on their website (www.perio.org).

The Periodontium

The teeth are composed of pulp, dentin and enamel. As mentioned in Chapter 3, the supporting tissues of the teeth are known as the periodontium and include cementum, periodontal ligament, bone and gingiva (Figure 9.1). The periodontal ligament suspends the teeth in the bony socket through a network of fibers which attach to the cementum of the root. The gingiva attaches to the bone via the periosteum and to the teeth through an attachment apparatus which has an epithelial component and a connective tissue component. This attachment is known as the "biologic width," and is an important factor when placing restorations near or under

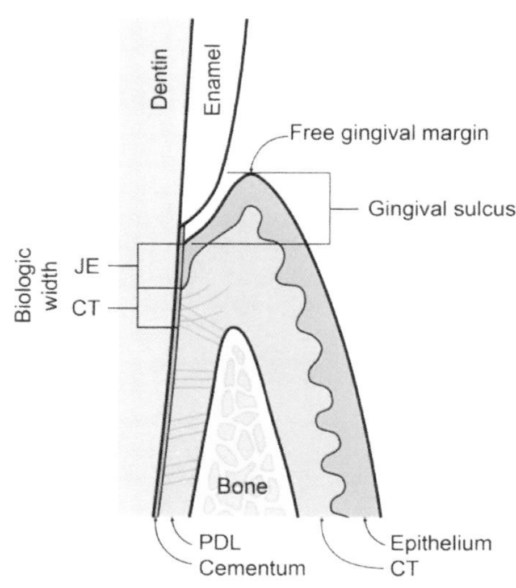

Figure 9.1 The periodontium consists of cementum, periodontal ligament (PDL) bone and the gingiva. JE = junctional epithelium, CT = connective tissue.

the gingival margin, as it can affect periodontal health. Above the attachment apparatus is free gingiva, which creates a gingival sulcus in between the tooth and the gingiva, commonly referred to by dentists as the periodontal "pocket". The depth of these pockets can be measured using a periodontal probe as an indicator of periodontal health. In health, periodontal pockets measure 0-3 mm in depth and can be maintained by patients with toothbrush and floss. For this reason periodontal probes are usually marked with alternating colors every 3 mm (Figure 9.2a).

Gingivitis

Gingivitis is a mild and reversible periodontal disease marked by gingival inflammation but no bone loss or soft tissue attachment loss. Visually, gingivitis presents with erythema (redness) and edema (swelling) of the gums. This often gives the gums a "rolled" edge instead of the "knife-edge" border found in healthy gingiva. Patients may also report pain or bleeding of the gums when they brush and floss. A good indicator of inflammation associated with gingivitis is prominent bleeding on probing (BOP) without an increase in probing depth.

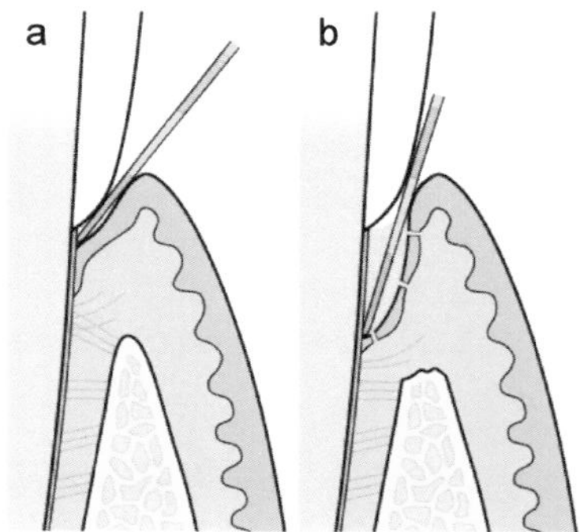

Figure 9.2 (a) A periodontal probe with 3mm increments is used to measure gingival pocket depths. (b) Periodontitis results in increased probing depths and/or loss of supporting bone and tissue attachment.

Periodontitis

Periodontitis is a more severe and destructive periodontal disease which presents with gingival attachment loss and/or bone loss. Gingival attachment loss measures 1-2mm in slight, 3-4mm in moderate and 5mm or more in severe periodontitis (9.2b). Radiographs are useful in assessing bone levels, which normally lie 1-2mm below the cementoenamel junction (CEJ). Bone loss is often estimated as a percentage of the root no longer covered by bone. For example, a range of 15-30% bone loss may be considered slight to moderate and greater than 30% is considered severe bone loss.

Bacterial Plaque and Calculus

Plaque is a natural bacterial biofilm that continuously forms on the surface of teeth. It is formed by colonizing bacteria in a matrix of salivary glycoproteins and extracellular polysaccharides adhering to the tooth and root surfaces. Plaque can be categorized as either supragingival or subgingival, and in most instances can be effectively removed by regular brushing and flossing. Over time, however, bacterial plaque hardens to become calculus, commonly referred to as tarter, which is mineralized plaque. Calculus (tarter) can only be effectively removed by a scaler. Scaling and root planing is required in deeper gingival pockets, where it is impossible for the bristles of a brush or floss to cleanse. Calculus is most prominently found on the lingual surfaces of mandibular anterior teeth and the buccal of maxillary posterior teeth, where the two major salivary ducts, the submandibular duct and parotid duct, respectively, bring minerals into the oral cavity via saliva.

Scaling and Root Planing

Due to the surgical nature of many periodontal therapies, the majority of a dental student's experience with periodontics is limited to scaling and root planing. Scaling and root planing is considered a part of initial periodontal therapy and may either be preparatory to surgical therapy or stand as definitive therapy. A combination of hand instruments and ultrasonic scalers is commonly used. Hand scalers, such as the Gracey curettes shown in Figure 9.3a, are used for various surfaces of the teeth and roots. For example, the Gracey 1/2 (one-two) is used for the mesial and distal surfaces of the anterior teeth, the 11/12 for the mesial surfaces of posterior teeth and the 13/14 is used for the distal surfaces of posterior teeth.

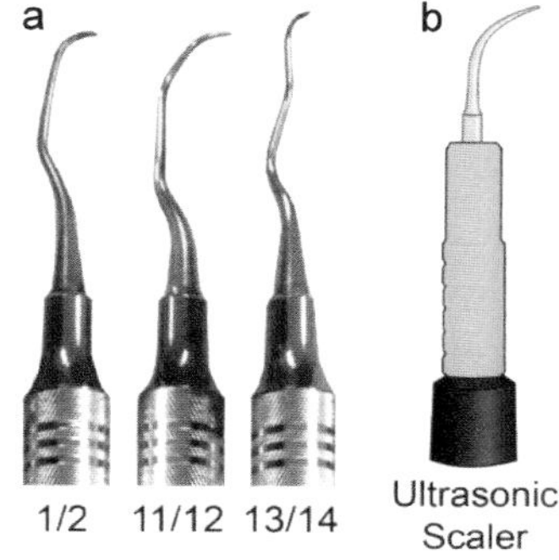

Figure 9.3 Plaque and calculus removal is commonly achieved using a combination of hand instruemtns such as the Gracey curettes (a) and ultrasonic scalers (b).

Ultrasonic scalers are electric instruments that are also used to remove plaque and calculus with water and small and fast vibrations at the tip of the instruments which results in either lateral or elliptical vibration, depending on the type of instrument selected (9.3b).

Periodontal surgery

Periodontists perform a wide variety of surgical procedures on the hard and soft tissues of the periodontium. Mucogingival surgeries may include gingivectomy, gingivoplasty, frenectomy (discussed in Chapter 10) and perio-plastic or esthetic surgeries. For example, certain anti-hypertensive and anti-epileptic medications increase the incidence of gingival overgrowth when coupled with poor oral hygiene (Figure 9.4a). A periodontist may perform a gingivectomy to remove excess gingiva coupled with gingivoplasty in order to reshape the gingiva and interdental papilla to recreate physiologic contours (9.4b).

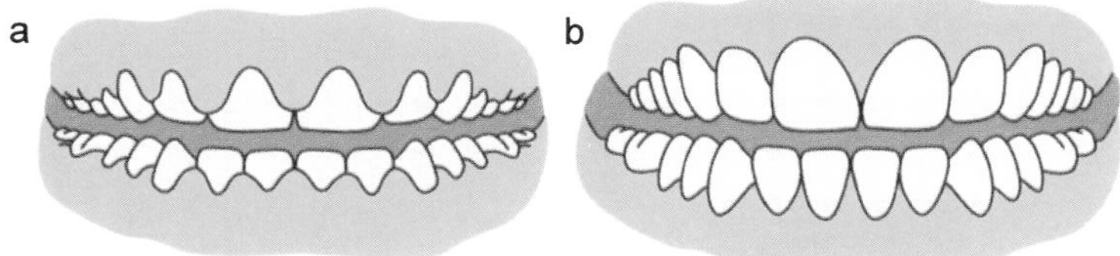

Figure 9.4 Gingival hyperplasia (a) can be surgically corrected with procedures known as gingivectomy and gingivoplasty to restore physiologic contours.

Osseous (bone) surgeries are also performed by periodontists and can be categorized as resective or regenerative. Resective osseous surgeries are performed to remove and recontour bone. Such surgeries can be performed to correct periodontal pockets and bony defects caused by periodontitis (Figure 9.5a). These pockets are impossible for a patient to clean, and very difficult for a dentist to scale due to lack of visibility and limited access under the gum tissue. A gingival flap can be reflected for direct access and more complete removal of subgingival plaque and calculus (9.5b, c).

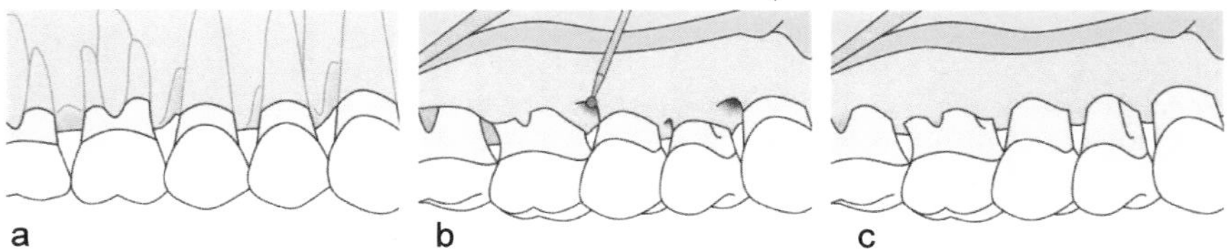

Figure 9.5 Periodontitis may cause deep periodontal pockets that require surgical intervention (a; the gingiva is not shown for clarity). The gingiva can be reflected to aid in access and visibility in order to debride the pockets. The bone can be reshaped to a more physiologically acceptable and cleansable contour.

Regenerative surgeries are done in order to add bone where it is deficient, such as repairing the above mentioned defects. Bone can also be grafted in preparation for implant placement where adequate bone volume is deficient, as adequate bone volume is crucial to successful implant placement. In addition, bone can be grafted into the tooth socket to preserve buccal bone when a tooth is extracted for a future implant site.

Implant Placement

Some dental schools incorporate implant restorations into their curriculum. Although an oral surgeon or periodontists will likely place the implant, the student may provide the surgeon with a surgical guide for implant placement and restore the implant with a crown. For example, a student may make a diagnostic alginate impression of the dental arches and pour the cast in stone (refer to Chapter 6). The student can then use the cast to orient the future placement of the implant based on the hard and soft tissues around the implant space and the desired position of the final crown. A surgical guide is fabricated from a resin material which houses a surgical sleeve that accurately orients the drill for the surgeon (Figure 9.4a). The apparatus is stabilized on the occlusal surfaces of adjacent teeth. A radiograph is made with the surgical guide in place in order to confirm the orientation of the surgical sleeve at an appointment called the “radiographic try-in” (9.4b). The surgeon can then utilize the guide to orient the drills and place the implant in the ideal location (9.4c,d).

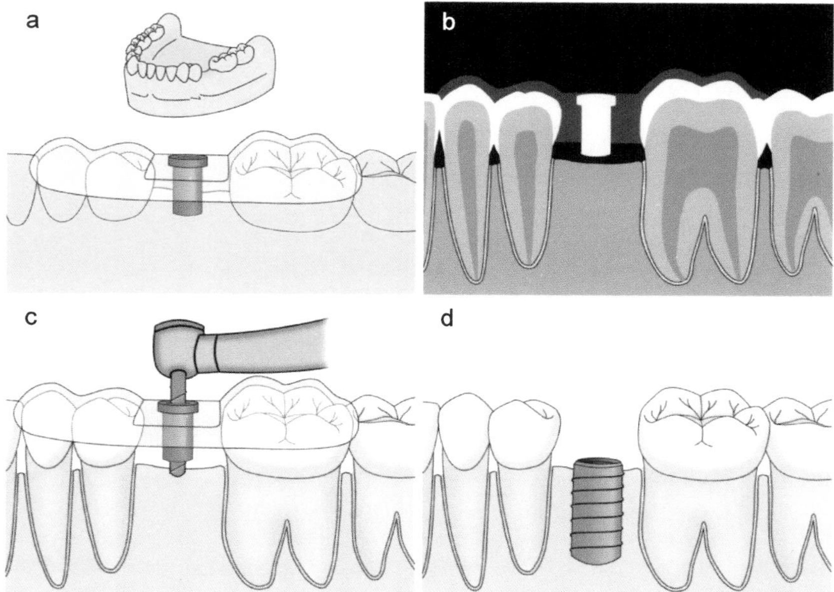

Figure 9.4 A diagnostic cast is poured in stone. From the cast, a surgical guide is fabricated to rest on the occlusal surfaces of adjacent teeth with a surgical sleeve insert (a). A radiographic image is taken with the surgical guide in the patient's mouth to assess the angulation (b). The surgical sleeve guides the surgeon's drill with copious irrigation to prevent overheating the bone (c). The implant is then placed into the void created by the drill (d).

Reviewed by
Dr. Paula Weistroffer, D.D.S., M.S.
Assistant Professor, Department of Periodontics
University of Iowa College of Dentistry

10

ORAL AND MAXILLOFACIAL SURGERY

Oral and maxillofacial surgery (OMFS) is the dental specialty that pertains to the diagnosis and surgical treatment of diseases, injuries and defects of the hard and soft tissues of the oral and maxillofacial region. The scope of oral surgery is vast, ranging from routine tooth extractions to facial reconstructions. An intimate knowledge of anatomy is required for this specialty, as many of the procedures deal directly with vital organs and structures. Oral surgery programs range from four to six years of post-graduate education, and some programs grant medical degrees (M.D.) upon their completion. More information can be found on the career and scope of oral surgery from the American Association of Oral and Maxillofacial Surgeons (AAOMS; www.aaoms.org).

Mandibular Anatomy and Anesthesia

The lower jaw is a single bone known as the mandible (Figure 10.1a). The body of the mandible houses the lower teeth in what is known as the alveolar process. The vertical portion of the mandible is known as the ramus, from which the condyles of the mandible project to articulate with the temporal bone of the skull. A nerve, known as the inferior alveolar nerve (IAN) enters the ramus of the mandible through the mandibular foramen. The lingual nerve, which provides sensation to the tongue and floor of the mouth, branches off from the IAN just before it enters the mandibular foramen. The IAN continues down through the ramus and to the body of the mandible through a canal, appropriately termed the inferior alveolar canal, and innervates each of the mandibular teeth by way of their apical foramina. An extension of the IAN known as the mental nerve also exits the body of the mandible through the mental foramen to provide sensation to the lower lip (10.1b). The IAN nerve also provides sensation to the lingual gingiva. A separate nerve, called the long buccal nerve, provides sensation to the gingiva facial to the lower teeth (not shown).

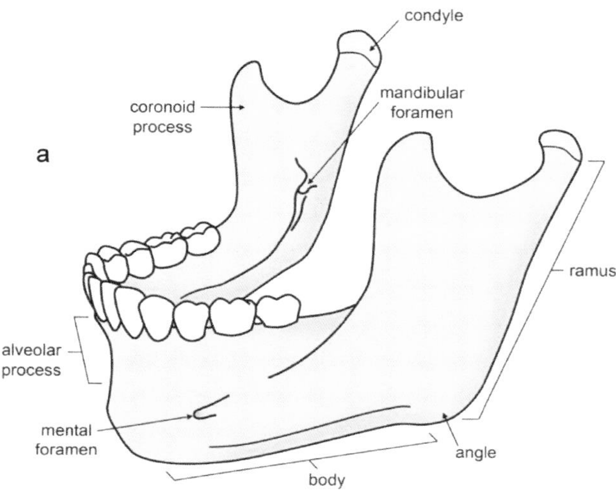

Figure 10.1 Anatomy of the mandible (a). Innervation of the mandibular teeth and lower jaw (b).

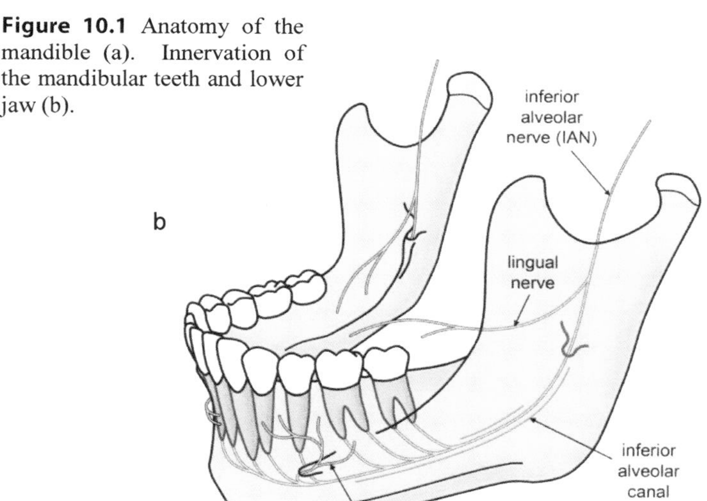

In general, an inferior alveolar nerve block is given to anesthetize the mandibular teeth. The target for this injection is just superior to the mandibular foramen in order to block the IAN as it enters the foramen into the inferior alveolar canal. When done correctly, an inferior alveolar nerve block anesthetizes all mandibular teeth on the side the anesthesia is administered, as well as the lingual gingiva and lower lip via the mental nerve. Due to the close proximity of the lingual nerve to the target area of the injection, the tongue is also commonly anesthetized on the side the injection is given. If you've ever had dental work done on your lower teeth, you may recall your tongue and lower lip being numb in addition to your teeth.

Maxillary Anatomy and Anesthesia

The upper jaw is also a single bone known as the maxilla (Figure 10.2a). The maxilla, as well as the mandible, actually begin as two separate bones that fuse together during development. However, the intermaxillary suture often remains more prominent than the suture in the mandible. The alveolar process of the maxilla houses the upper teeth. The maxilla articulates with many bones of the skull, after which several parts of the maxilla can be named e.g. the zygomatic process of the maxilla articulates with the zygomatic bone, the frontal process with the frontal bone, etc. Several different nerves innervate the maxillary teeth, conveniently named the posterior, middle and anterior superior alveolar nerves, which innervate the molars, premolars and anterior teeth, respectively. The infraorbital nerve extends to exit the maxilla through the infraorbital foramen just under each orbital rim. The infraorbital nerve branches into the inferior palpebral, external nasal and superior labial nerves. These three supply the lower eyelid, ala of the nose and upper lip, respectively (10.2b). The hard palate is innervated mainly by the greater palatine and the nasopalatine nerves (not shown).

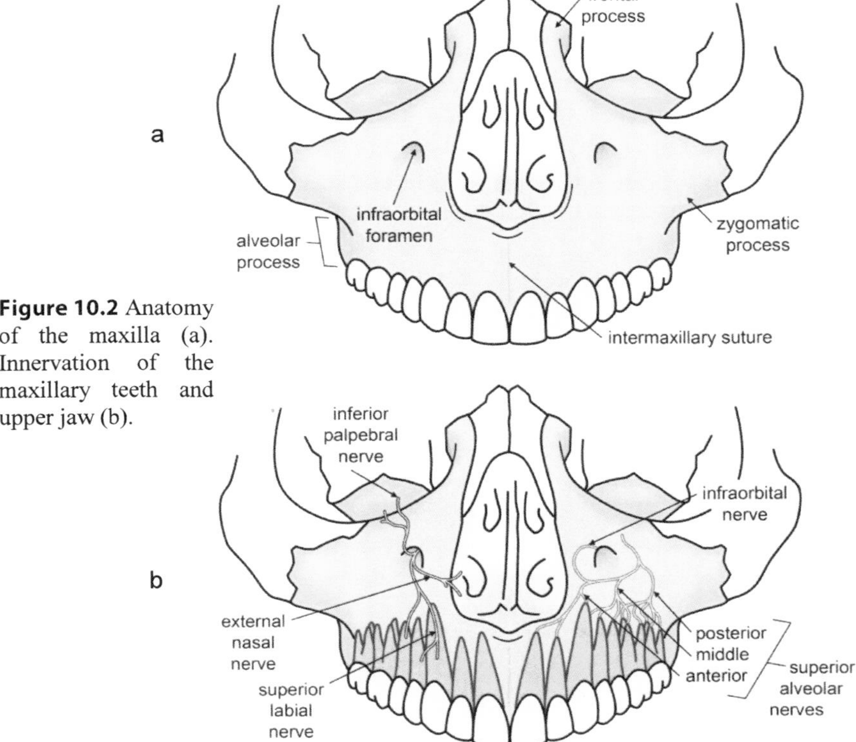

Figure 10.2 Anatomy of the maxilla (a). Innervation of the maxillary teeth and upper jaw (b).

Anesthesia for maxillary teeth may be given on a per-tooth basis or via nerve blocks. When working on one or several adjacent teeth, a local infiltration injection may be given. This is done by placing the needle tip in close proximity to the maxilla at a level just higher than the apex of the target tooth. Local anesthetic easily dissolves through the buccal plate of the maxilla to reach the nerve(s) underneath. Due to the close proximity of the infraorbital nerve to the middle superior nerve and the apices of the canine and first premolar, the infraorbital nerve is often also anesthetized when numbing these areas. If you've ever had dental work done in this area, you may remember a heavy eyelid, a tingly nostril and a puffy lip. Palatal injections are also given as needed when the lingual gingiva may be affected during treatment.

Simple Tooth Extractions

Teeth may be extracted for a number of reasons – severe caries, periodontal disease, impaction, infection, as part of orthodontic treatment, or prior to prosthetic treatment – to name a few. There are also many instruments and techniques that can be used to extract a given tooth, many of which are made for specific types of teeth. In general, the soft tissue attachment is first released from the tooth with periosteal elevators. Next, the tooth is elevated or displaced from the surrounding bone with a dental elevator. These preparatory steps indicate pronounced anesthesia and allow for more apical positioning of extraction forceps. The beaks of the forceps are then placed on the tooth to be extracted and the tooth is luxated in an apical, buccal and lingual direction using slow, steady forces. For teeth with a conical root, rotational forces may also be applied prior to extraction (Figure 10.3). Smaller elevators and picks are used to remove portions of the root(s) that remain in the socket (not shown).

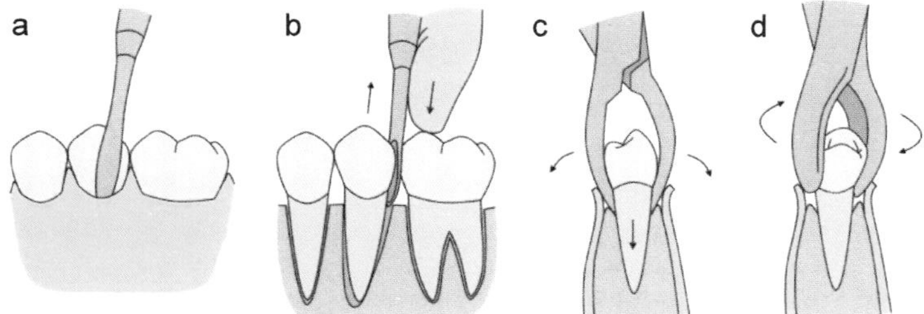

Figure 10.3 Simple tooth extraction involves loosening the soft tissue attachment from the tooth (a), luxating the tooth in its socket (b) and applying buccal, lingual and apical forces to the tooth (c). Rotational forces may also be applied in the tooth has a conical root form (d).

Pre-Prosthetic Surgery

Edentulous ridges must meet certain morphologic criteria in order for a removable prosthesis to function properly and provide ideal retention and stability. Often times, when extracting teeth, an avleoloplasty is performed in addition to the extractions in order to remove bony undercuts and help shape the remaining edentulous ridge in preparation for denture fabrication (Figure 10.4).

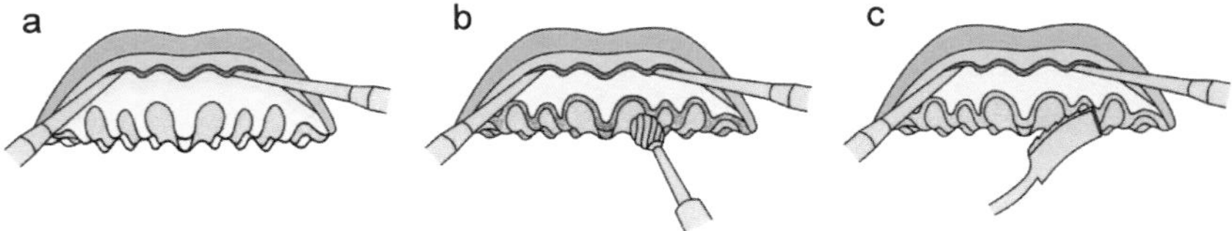

Figure 10.4 Alveoloplasty involves retracting the gingival tissues (a), removing and recontouring interproximal bone (b) and smoothing the resulting bone for a free-flowing finish (c).

Bony swellings known as exostoses or tori are quite common in the general population and tend to occur in the palate (torus palatinus) and mandible lingual to the premolar area (torus mandibularis). Removal of these bony growths may be indicated prior to fabricating a maxillary or mandibular removable prosthesis. Figure 10.5 shows one technique for mandibular tori removal, first by creating a moat around the torus with a bur, then dislodging it with a chisel.

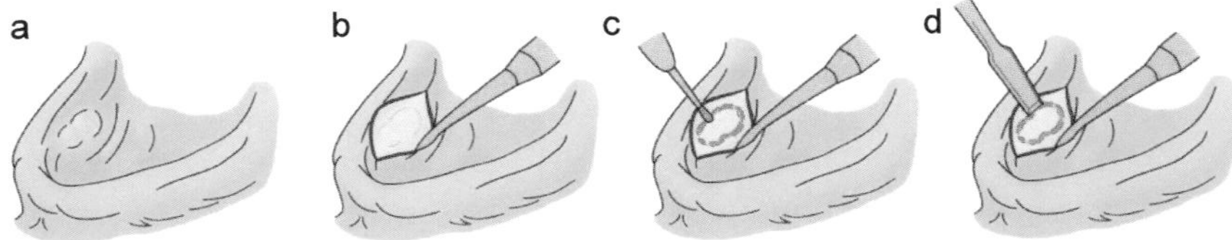

Figure 10.5 Mandibular tori (a) are first exposed with a gingival flap (b). The borders of the tori are then accentuated with a bur (c) and chiseled off (d).

Soft tissues can also interfere with removable prosthetics. A frenum is a thin band of fibrous connective tissue that connects muscle fibers of the lip or cheek to the periosteum of the alveolar ridges. When this attachment is high on the ridge, it can act to dislodge a denture, and excision may be necessary. A simple excision along the lateral margins of the frenum to the periosteum may suffice with sutures to close the resulting wound (Figure 10.6).

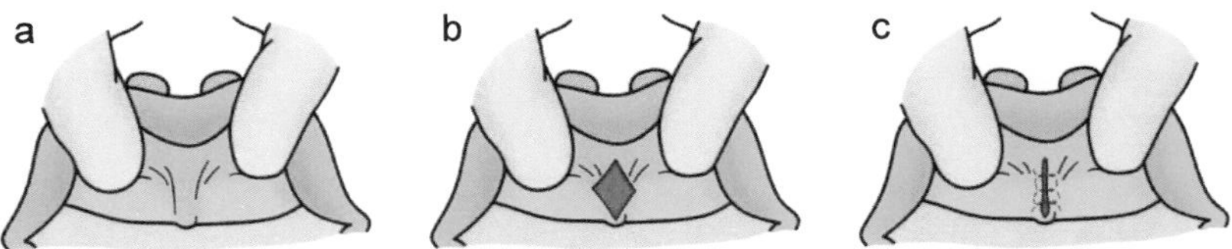

Figure 10.6 A labial frenum can act to dislodge removable prostheses if the attachment is high on the ridge (a). A simple excision along the lateral margins of the frenum (b) with sutures can produce a favorable result (c).

Other Aspects of Oral Surgery

Aside from extractions and pre-prosthetic surgeries, oral surgeons provide a wide variety of treatments to patients and often coordinate treatment with general practitioners, other dental specialties or medical doctors. Oral surgeons are trained to manage complex maxillofacial traumas and oral and facial lesions and infections. Implant placement (discussed in Chapter 9) and surgical intervention of temporomandibular joint (TMJ) disorders are also performed by oral surgeons. Orthognathic surgeries and treatment of congenital deformities, such as cleft lip and palate, require the expertise of an oral surgeon. Advanced surgeries are beyond the scope of this book, however orthognathic surgeries are briefly discussed simply to provide a glimpse into the possibilities of modern surgical techniques.

Orthognathic Surgery

Orthognathic surgery refers to a surgical-orthodontic treatment program used to achieve a stable dentoskeletal relationship in the context of facial balance and esthetics. Orthognathic surgery may be considered for patients whose skeletal discrepancy cannot be effectively and/or esthetically compensated by orthodontic tooth movement alone. The surgeries mentioned in this section will likely only be experienced during a dental school curriculum in the form of observing or assisting an oral surgeon.

Mandibular and maxillary osteotomies are performed in order to change the location or appearance of the jaws. The bilateral sagittal split osteotomy (BSSO) is commonly used to set back or advance the mandible forward. In this technique, the surgeon makes a transoral incision that displaces the ramus and posterior body of the mandible sagittally, which allows repositioning of the anterior portion of the mandible. This allows the clinician the freedom to reposition the mandible in a way that promotes healing by maintaining bony contact. Rigid internal fixation devices such as screws and plates are then used to stabilize the pieces of the mandible together (Figure 10.7).

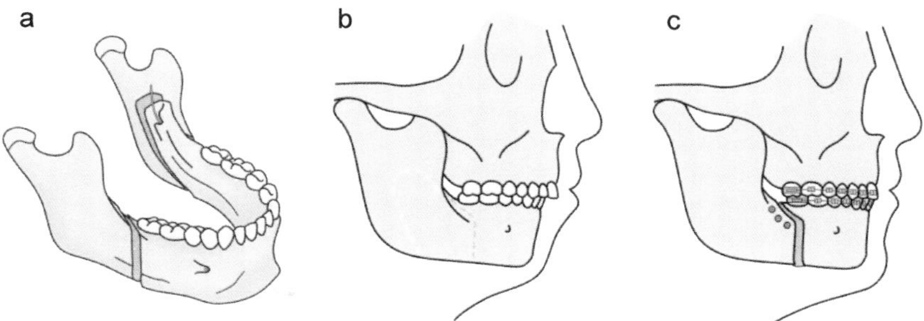

Figure 10.7 The bilateral sagittal split osteotomy (BSSO) makes two separate incisions (a) to move the anterior potion of the mandible forward and fix it in this new position (b, c).

A genioplasty is commonly used to modify the inferior border of the mandible and can be done either alone or in conjunction with mandibular osteotomy as a means make an ineffective chin more pronounced. The cut for a genioplasty is made anterior to the mental foramen in order to avoid the mental nerve. The anterior portion is then secured in the desired position with a fixation device such as a screw (Figure 10.8).

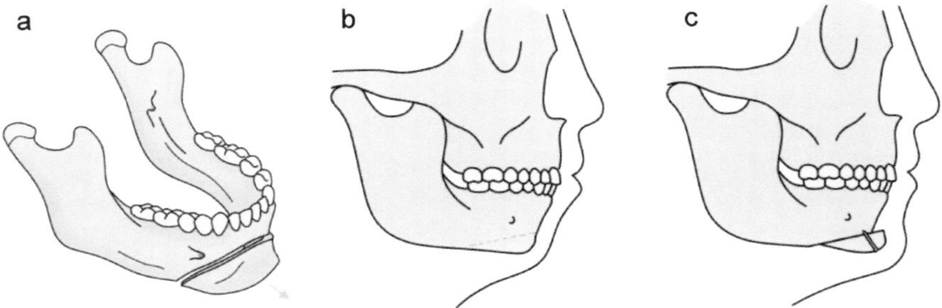

Figure 10.8 A genioplasty can be used to treat an insufficient chin without changing occlusion (a, b, c). It is a relatively simpler procedure that may be used in conjunction with other orthognathic treatments.

Maxillary deformities can also be modified by orthognathic means. For example, a maxillary deficiency may be evidenced by a mid-facial concavity on a profile view. A procedure known as a Le Fort I advancement may be performed to correct this deficiency. The surgeon first sections the maxilla to free the alveolar process, moves it into a more favorable position and secures it into position with plates and screws (Figure 10.9).

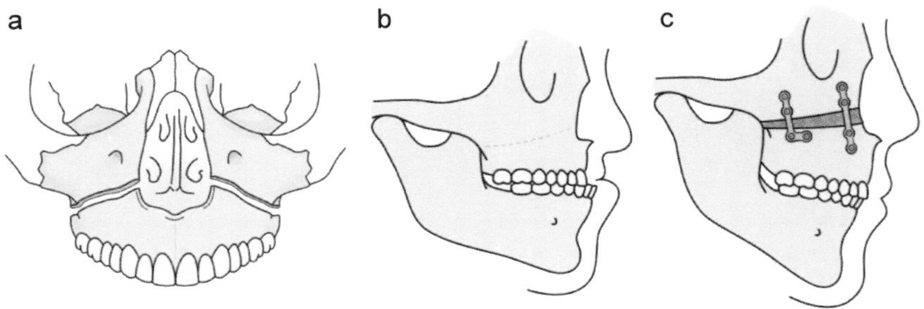

Figure 10.9 A Le Fort I advancement (a) allows alterations to the position of the maxillary, commonly used to correct maxillary deficiency (b). The maxilla is secured into position with plates and screws (c).

11

ENDODONTICS

Endodontics ("endo" for short) is the branch of dentistry which is concerned with the dental pulp and the periradicular tissues, or tissues surrounding the roots of teeth. Endodontists are commonly known as "root canal specialists" because root canal therapy is the most common treatment they provide. Endodontists perform an average of 25 root canal treatments per week, whereas general dentists perform around two.[6] There are currently 55 advanced specialty programs in endodontics in the U.S. and Canada. More information about the specialty can be obtained from the American Association of Endodontists (www.aae.org).

Tooth Roots and Pulp Cavities

Like the iceberg that sunk the Titanic, much of a tooth's anatomy is hidden under a sea of bone and gingiva. Endodontists as well as general practitioners performing endodontic treatment must have an intimate knowledge of root morphology and internal anatomy. In addition to knowing "normal" anatomy, dentists must also be aware of common variations in order to locate and safely treat all canals in a diseased tooth. A major cause of endodontic failure is the inability to locate, chemomechanically clean and properly fill all canals in the root canal system. Throughout your dental program you will be asked to memorize anatomical variations for each tooth. For the time being, a brief study of the most common anatomy is appropriate, upon which variations and details can be added in dental school (Figure 11.1).

Maxillary anterior teeth usually have one root with one canal inside. Maxillary first premolars are unique in that they usually have two roots – a buccal root and a lingual root – and two canals, one in each root. Maxillary second premolars present with one root and either one or two canals. Maxillary first

---

[6] "Endododontic Facts." American Association of Endodontists. Web. Jan. 2012. <http://www.aae.org>.

molars usually have three roots and four canals. Their root system consists of two buccal roots and one lingual/palatal root. The distobuccal and lingual roots each contain one canal while the mesiobuccal root usually contains two canals, referred to as MB and MB_2. Maxillary second molars also have three roots and may or may not present with an MB_2. Maxillary third molars commonly have three fused roots although their morphology is quite variable in nature and root canal therapy is not commonly performed on third molars.

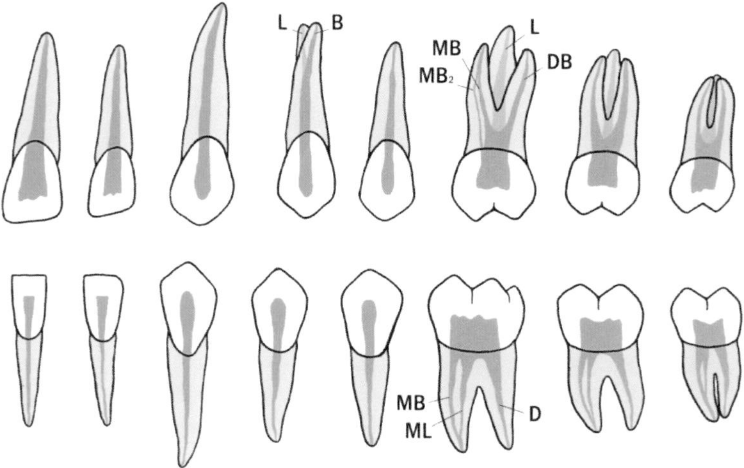

Figure 11.1 The most common root and pulp morphology of the teeth.

Mandibular anterior teeth and premolars most commonly present with one root and one canal, although it is not uncommon for these teeth to contain two canals or two roots, one buccal and one lingual. Mandibular molars present with two roots, one mesial and one distal. Mandibular molars usually contain either three or four canals, two in the mesial root and either one or two in the distal root. Mandibular third molars, like maxillary third molars, are variable in morphology but commonly have two fused roots.

Pulpal Pathosis

As mentioned in Chapter 3, the dental pulp is a living tissue containing blood vessels and sensory nerves. Like most living tissue, irritation of the pulp results in cell death and inflammation proportional to the severity and intensity of tissue damage. The most common irritants to dental pulp are microorganisms as caries gets closer and closer to the pulp. Even small carious lesions are capable of eliciting a pulpal response by producing toxins which can penetrate the pulp through dentinal tubules.[7] Other irritants to the pulp include mechanical, chemical

7 Brannstrom M, Lind P: Pulpal response to early dental caries, Journal of Dental Research 44:1045, 1965.

and thermal irritants. For example, trauma may cause a longitudinal tooth fracture which can act as a reservoir for microorganisms and allow their progression to the pulp and cause inflammation.

Moderate to severe pulpal injuries propagate additional immune responses and cause a higher concentration of inflammatory mediators to be released. Due to the confinement of the dental pulp within the dentin, the pulp is unable to expand or swell during inflammation, resulting in an increase in tissue pressure. This pressure is sensed by the nerve endings within the pulp and interpreted as pain. The increased tissue pressure coupled with a decrease in blood circulation can result in pulpal necrosis and periradicular pathosis. Figure 11.2 summarizes a typical sequence in pulpal and periradicular pathosis.

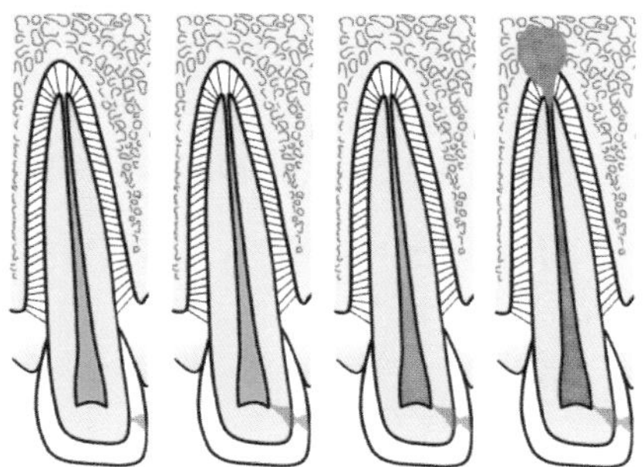

Figure 11.2 A typical sequence by which caries may penetrate the pulp and periapical tissues.

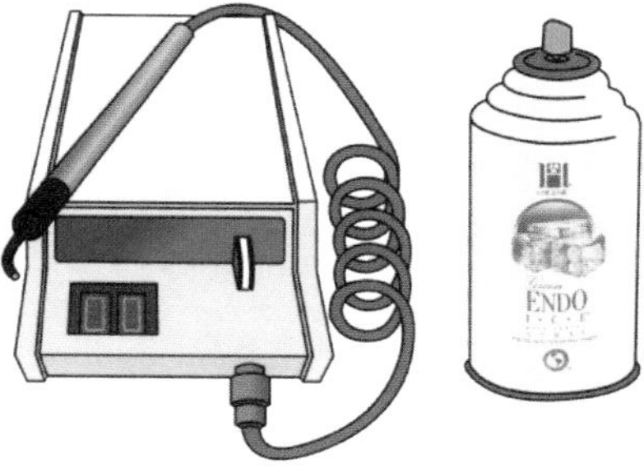

Figure 11.3 Common pulpal tests include electronic pulp testing (left) and refrigerant sprays (right).

Classification of Pulpal Diseases

Diagnosis and classification of pulpal conditions is usually based on subjective and objective clinical symptoms and radiographic images. A subjective evaluation may include questioning the patient to determine the severity and nature of pain while objective testing is done in an attempt to reproduce the pain and assess the patient's symptoms. Radiographic images allow the dentist to assess the extent of the infection and its effects on the periapical tissues. A brief description of the most common classification of pulpal conditions is given.

Normal Pulp

A normal tooth will exhibit no clinical symptoms and be responsive to vitality tests. Various tests are used to assess tooth vitality, such as electrical pulp testing (EPT) and cold tests. Electrical pulp testers produce an electrical current and transmit electricity to a tooth through a conductive medium, usually toothpaste. The patient completes the circuit by holding onto the handle of the instrument and lets go to break the circuit when they start to feel the tooth tingle. The cold test can be done using a refrigerant spray on a cotton to stimulate a tooth. Teeth with vital pulps respond positively to electrical stimuli and present with a sharp pain to cold stimuli that goes away once the stimulus is removed (Figure

11.3). Teeth that do not respond to or cannot sense either the electric or cold stimulus may be deemed necrotic, or "dead".

Reversible Pulpitis

Reversible pulpitis is a condition in which either caries is present or the dentin is exposed, causing a response from the pulp. In reversible pulpitis, removing the caries and covering the exposed dentin with a restoration will prevent further pulpal insult and allow it to heal properly.

Symptomatic Irreversible Pulpitis

Irreversible pulpitis results when caries progresses very close to or enters the pulp chamber or when a traumatic injury fractures a tooth to expose the pulp. In cases of irreversible pulpitis, the pulp is affected to an extent that it will not recover, and thus root canal treatment is indicated.

A tooth with symptomatic irreversible pulpitis will test positive to EPT and cold tests. However, instead of a short, sharp pain upon thermal stimulation, the tooth will present with a lingering pain that remains well after the stimulus is removed.

Asymptomatic Irreversible Pulpitis

Occasionally teeth with deep caries respond normally to cold and EPT tests but radiographically appear to approximate the pulp chamber. In these situations caries excavation is needed to determine whether caries has reached the pulp. If complete caries removal can be performed without exposing the pulp, a restoration may be placed and a diagnosis of reversible pulpitis can be made. If caries excavation leads to a pulpal exposure, a diagnosis of asymptomatic irreversible pulpitis can be made and root canal treatment may be initiated.

Pulpal Necrosis

Pulpal necrosis is the technical term for a "dead tooth". Teeth with pulpal necrosis may also be referred to as "non-vital" teeth. When necrosis occurs, the pulpal tissues are replaced with bacteria, inflammatory cells and debris. Pulpal necrosis may result either from a deep carious lesion or from traumatic injury which either exposes the pulp or displaces the tooth so that its blood supply is severed. A tooth with pulpal necrosis will not respond to either EPT or cold stimulation and may show radiographic changes at the tip of the root consistent with bone loss as a result of chronic inflammation.

Principles of Root Canal Therapy

Root canal therapy is commonly performed in order to maintain a natural tooth as opposed to extraction and replacement with a bridge or implant. In its most basic form, the goal of root canal treatment is to remove pulpal tissue and any bacterial debris that may have penetrated the pulpal cavity. Canals are then shaped in order to facilitate filling them with a rubbery material known as gutta percha.

A pre-operative radiograph is made in order to diagnose disease, allow for measurement of tooth length and assess case difficulty. For example, a dark (radiolucent) circle at the apex of a root with an apparent carious etiology indicates pulpal necrosis with an infection that has progressed through the pulp and into the surrounding bone. A pre-operative radiograph can also provide initial dimensions of a tooth. The total length of the tooth is an important factor to consider when first instrumenting the canals (Figure 11.4). It is common for the apical foramen to be around 1mm short of the end of the root. For this reason, most instrumentation is performed short of total length as visualized on the radiograph. Case difficulty is also considered by general dentists as a guide for when to refer to an endodontic specialist.

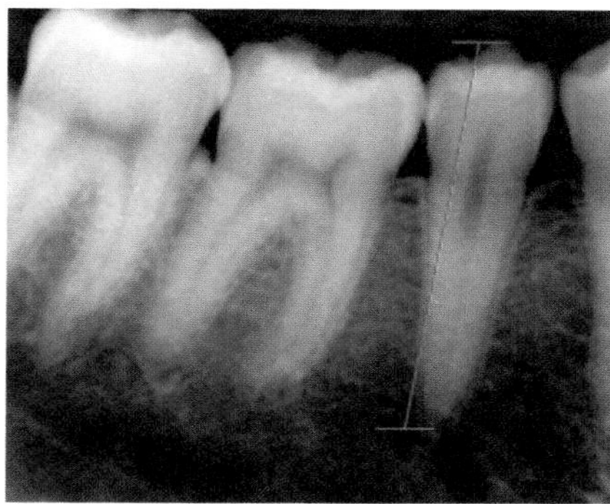

Figure11.4 A pre-operative radiograph allows for an assessment of the periapex and initial measurements, such total tooth length.

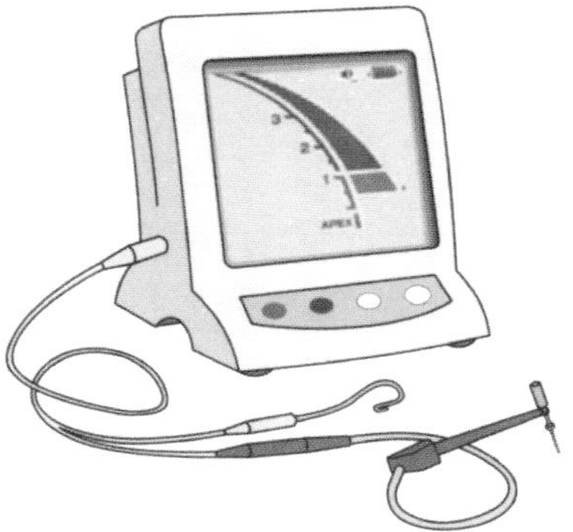

Figure 11.5 An apex locator uses frequencies of alternating current to determine the length of canals.

While many restorative dental procedures avoid the pulp at all costs, endodontists drill specifically to reach the pulp during root canal therapy for what is known as the access preparation. An access preparation is an opening into the lingual (anterior teeth) or occlusal surface (posterior teeth) which conserves as much tooth structure as possible while exposing the entire pulp chamber, allowing access to the canals (Figure 11.6a,b). The length of the canals may be determined either by taking a "working length" radiograph with files in each of the canals or, more commonly, using a machine known as an apex locator to locate the apical limits of the canal system (Figure 11.5).

Canals are then instrumented with stainless steel hand files and/or nickel titanium rotary instruments to the proper working length (11.6c). All pulpal tissue and bacterial debris must be cleaned from the canals with increasingly larger files. The canals must also be shaped with the files to a continuous tapered form from the orifice to the apex of each canal. This creates a canal with smooth walls and facilitates their filling with gutta percha material. A gutta percha point known as a master cone (MC) is fitted to match the diameter of the apical extent of the root canal preparation and seal the apex (11.6d). Additional gutta percha is added in order to completely fill the canal, a process known as obturation, which completes root canal treatment (11.6e).

The dentist must decide what type of restoration is appropriate for the tooth depending on several factors, such as how much tooth structure remains after caries removal and root canal therapy. In our animated example, a foundation and a crown were placed in order to return the tooth to normal form and function (11.6f). The definitive restoration provides the coronal seal. Together with the master cone, the canal system of the tooth is now sealed from the oral environment.

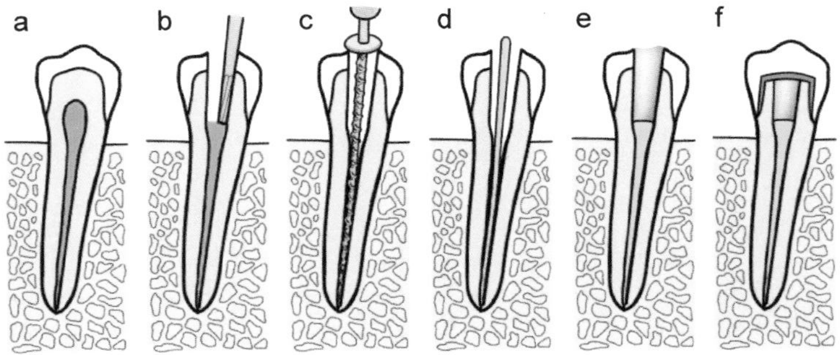

Figure 11.6 Root canal treatment begins with an access opening into the pulp chamber (a, b). Next, next the canal is cleaned and shaped with hand files or rotary instruments (c). The canal is then obturated with gutta percha (d). The chamber of the pulp cavity is then restored with either a temporary or permanent restoration (e). The restoration may also act as a foundation for a crown (f).

Reviewed by
Dr. Robert Beasley, D.M.D.
Resident, Department of Endodontics
University of Iowa College of Dentistry

ABOUT THE AUTHOR

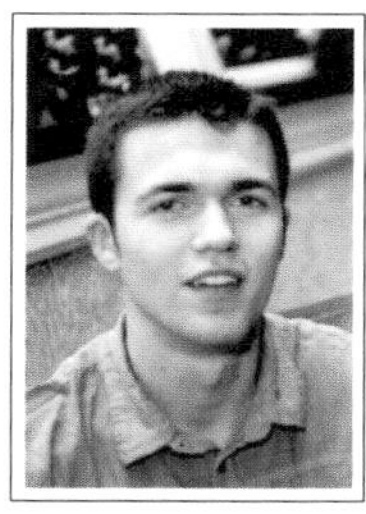

John Syrbu was born in Chisinau, Moldova. At the age of 5, his family moved to Farmington, CT and then to Iowa City, IA when he was 11. John currently resides in Iowa City where he attends the University of Iowa College of Dentistry as a third year dental student. He lives with his fiancé, Natalie (also a third year dental student) and the two of them enjoy adventure and travel, going to the gym and cooking at home.

In addition to illustrating the images for this book, John draws dental cartoons which are published in the national dental student newsletter, *ASDA News*, and posted to a Facebook page he created called "Dental Art and Humor". He is also currently authoring and illustrating electronic children's books in order to encourage and establish good oral hygiene habits for young children. John hopes to be able to continue developing his passion for dentistry through art and writing.

Made in the USA
Charleston, SC
10 April 2012